MCQs on Clinical Pharmacology

D0346045

MCQs on Clinical Pharmacology

D.R. Laurence MD FRCP
Professor Emeritus of Pharmacology and Therapeutics,
School of Medicine,
University College, London

P.N. Bennett MD FRCP
Consultant Physician,
Royal United Hospital, Bath
and Senior Lecturer in Clinical Pharmacology,
University of Bath

J.F. Stokes MD FRCP
Consulting Physician,
University College Hospital, London

SECOND EDITION

Churchill Livingstone
EDINBURGH LONDON MELBOURNE AND NEW YORK 1988

CHURCHILL LIVINGSTONE
Medical Division of Longman Group Limited

Distributed in the United States of America by Churchill
Livingstone Inc., 650 Avenue of the Americas, New York,
N.Y. 10011, and by associated companies, branches and
representatives throughout the world.

First edited 1983
Second edition 1988
  Reprinted 1992
  Reprinted 1993
  Reprinted 1994

ISBN 0 443 03416 8

British Library Cataloguing in Publication Data
A catalogue record for this book is available from the British Library

Library of Congress Cataloging in Publication Data
Laurence, D.R. (Desmond Roger)
  MCQs on clinical pharmacology.
  "Questions based on Clinical Pharmacology (6th
  edition) by D.R. Laurence and P.N. Bennett"–Pref.
  1. Pharmacology–Examinations, questions, etc.
  I. Bennett, P.N.   II. Stokes, J.F. (John Fisher)
  III. Laurence, D.R. (Desmond Roger). Clinical
  pharmacology.   IV. Title
  RM301.13.L38   1988   615'.1076   88-9534

The
publisher's
policy is to use
**paper manufactured
from sustainable forests**

Produced by Longman Singapore Publishers (Pte) Ltd
Printed in Singapore

Preface

This is a book of multiple choice questions based on *Clinical Pharmacology* (6th edition) by D.R. Laurence and P.N. Bennett. Its objective is to help medical students and postgraduates to pass examinations in clinical pharmacology.

We are, in principle, in favour of such examinations because we think knowledge of drugs and medicines is essential to the competent practice of medicine. Patients are entitled to expect competence from their physician, and physicians owe to their patients a duty of care.

To answer questions is the surest way of finding out whether you know a subject. That some examinations and questions are ill-suited to their purpose does not nullify the principle. *The easiest and the best way to pass an examination is to know its subject.*

It is too easy to read a book and to assume that this has been a profitable exertion. But too often it has not been so. The best assurance that reading has been profitable is to be required or to require oneself to *use* what has been read.

A convenient, quick and private way of doing this is to test yourself with multiple choice questions. Errors teach, if it is possible at once to verify them in an appropriate text; otherwise frustration is the result.

Although *more experienced users* may attempt the questions as they stand, with the object of testing the range of their knowledge, *less experienced* may prefer to read a chapter of the book, and after an interval of some hours, try to answer the questions in this volume. Wrong choices are best checked with the book as they are made, since the purpose is to learn, not merely to record a score.

In almost all cases the correct answer will be found either explicitly or by obvious implication in the text of the chapter being studied, but occasionally reference to another chapter will be needed. Drugs may feature in more than one chapter (eg β-adrenoceptor blocking agents) and, when a principle of pharmacokinetics or an adverse reaction is involved, chapters 8 and 9 will repay study. Use of the index is seldom needed, though educationally it is no bad thing to have to search beyond a single chapter for an answer.

Some of the questions are inevitably based on simple memory of facts, the building blocks of pharmacology and medicine. But, in producing these questions we have tried not only to inform and remind but also to illustrate principles. It will be found, therefore, that many apparently factual questions can be answered from knowledge of principles. (Principle = fundamental truth as a basis for reasoning: OED.)

Questions are all of the familiar multiple True/False type in which any number of choices within each question may be correct.

1988   DRL, PNB, JFS

Contents

1 Topics in Drug Therapy and Clinical Pharmacology

1.1 In drug therapy, the following statements are correct:

A Efficacy and safety of a drug lie solely in its chemical nature
B Considerations of pharmacokinetics are important
C Drugs are the major causative factor in the decline of mortality from infectious diseases of the past 100 years
D The concept of benefit versus risk is central to proper practice
E Whenever a drug is given a risk is taken

1.2 Disease may be

A cured by a course of a drug
B suppressed or controlled, without cure, by a drug
C prevented by a drug
D worsened by a drug
E mimicked by a drug

1.3 Iatrogenic disease

A occurs as a result of self-medication
B occurs as a result of prescribed medication
C is far from rare
D may result from bad medical advice
E may be the result of patient non-compliance with clear instructions

1.4   Risk

A   may be graded as unacceptable, acceptable or negligible

B   involved in using penicillin is such that it should only be used in life-endangering infections

C   if unnecessary, is avoided by most people in their daily lives

D   is ignored by most people if it is less than 1:100 000

E   of death from a drug contraindicates its use

1.5   Modern synthetic drugs

A   should not be used until a firm aetiological diagnosis has been made

B   benefit the quality of life more than they do its quantity (duration)

C   are toxic because they are synthetic, not natural, chemicals

D   can only be evaluated by strict randomised controlled trials

E   are only acceptable for use in therapeutics if their mode of action is known

1.6   The following statements about non-scientific, unorthodox medical systems and traditional medicine are correct:

A   Of the terms alternative, fringe and complementary medicine, the term complementary is preferred

B   Traditional or indigenous (pre-scientific) medical systems have provided no drugs that have stood the test of scientific evaluation

C   Beliefs that cannot be disproved by scientific testing are a feature of unorthodox medical systems

D   Scientific evaluation of unorthodox medical systems is inherently impracticable

E   Iatrogenic disease does not occur in traditional medicine

1.7 **The following statements comply with homoeopathic beliefs or practice:**

A Only one disease can exist in the body at any one time

B Natural disease is cured by introducing into the body by means of a medicine, an artificial disease, which drives out the natural disease

C The effects of drugs are potentiated by dilution provided each dose contains at least one molecule of drug

D By shaking a medicine correctly a spiritual therapeutic energy is released

E If homoeopathic principles (beliefs) cannot be substantiated, ie tested and confirmed by use of scientific method, then homoeopathic treatments cannot work

1.8 **The following statements about the hazards of life on drugs are correct:**

A Risk of adverse effects increases continuously with duration of drug therapy

B Homeostatic physiological mechanisms add to the efficacy of drugs

C Prolonged administration of a receptor agonist induces up-regulation of receptors

D Changes in receptors can explain both tolerance to continuing administration of a drug and rebound effects on abrupt withdrawal

E Chronic drug use may make patients more vulnerable to intercurrent illness

1.9 **The following statements about liability for adverse effects of drugs are correct:**

A Liability to compensate for injury of another person caused by negligence (fault) is usual in all legal systems

B If a patient suffers an adverse drug reaction, someone (the producer or prescriber, for instance) has been negligent

C It is easy to determine whether an adverse event or worsening of health is due to a drug

D Some adverse drug reactions could as readily be said to be due to a 'defect' in the patient as to a 'defect' in the drug

E Capacity to cause harm is inherent in even the most useful drugs

1.10 **Despite the manifest difficulties of providing special compensation for drug-caused injury, a scheme to meet public demand might be found socially and politically acceptable if it incorporated the following concepts:**

A Liability for drugs under trial before being licenced for general use should fall on the producer

B Liability for recently licenced (by an official regulatory body) drugs may reasonably be shared between the producer and the community (government)

C Liability for standard drugs should fall on a central fund

D Compensation in the case of standard drugs should only be for rare serious effects not ordinarily taken into account when prescribing the drug

E Prolonged legal argument may have to be accepted in cases of compensation for the effects of standard drugs

1.11 **The following statements about warnings to patients are correct:**

A Doctors do no more than frighten patients by warning them of adverse effects of drugs

B Doctors have a legal duty to warn patients of risks to the extent that in the doctors' judgement is compatible with the particular patient's welfare

C If patients experience adverse reactions of which they were not warned then doctors will be convicted of negligence

D Since patients have died of the consequences of venepuncture, anyone asked to undergo the procedure should be told this fact before deciding whether to agree

E If a patient expresses a wish to leave all considerations of risks of treatment to the doctor, the doctor should yet insist on telling the patient of these risks

1.12 **Drug therapy carries risk**

A because drugs are not sufficiently selective

B which has been reduced by the development of target-selective carriers such as antibodies

C because patients are homogeneous

D because patients unpredictably develop allergy to drugs

E because dosage adjustment is unavoidably imprecise

1.13 **When taking a patient's history special enquiry should be made about previous use of medicines or other drugs because**

A drugs can cause disease
B withdrawal of drugs can cause disease
C drugs can interact with each other
D drugs can leave residual effects after administration and withdrawal
E knowledge of drug history assists choice of medication in the future

1.14 **Repeat prescriptions in general practice (primary care) are provided by doctors**

A only after personal discussion with the patient
B as a way of getting rid of a patient
C as a way of maintaining a relationship
D when they cannot think of anything better to do
E for a patient whose health depends on the specific pharmacological effect of the drug

1.15 **The following statements or opinions about economics in medicine are correct:**

A There are two countries in the world that have enough resources to meet all their citizens' demands for medical care
B Health care cannot be rationed and attempts to do so should not be made
C Cost-effectiveness analysis is a broader activity than is cost-benefit analysis
D Doctors should think only of their patients' immediate personal needs, should fight for these and should not allow economic considerations to intrude
E All expenditure of resources carries a cost in benefits foregone elsewhere, ie 'opportunity cost'

1.16 The following statements about drug therapy are correct:

A The response in acute infections is much influenced by the interaction of the personalities of doctor and patient

B The response in anxiety or depression is primarily determined by the choice of drug and has little to do with the personal interaction of doctor, patient and social environment

C Response to a drug can be significantly affected by the initial level of activity of the target organ or system

D It is of no consequence what sort of medicine the patient thinks he has been given, all that matters is what he has in fact been given

E Knowledge of *why* a patient gets better is of purely academic interest

1.17 A placebo effect

A may follow treatment of all kinds

B only occurs in mentally ill patients

C in the individual is an inconstant attribute

D can be expected in about 35% of patients

E following a tonic usually has a distinct pharmacological basis

1.18 Placebo reactors tend to be

A introverted

B unsociable

C acquiescent

D lacking in self-confidence

E neurotic

1.19 The quality of life of a patient can be assessed by using questionnaires that record, amongst other things,

A sleep

B physical mobility

C energy

D pain

E emotional reactions

1.20 **Factors established as being associated with patient non-compliance include**

A   lack of understanding of instructions
B   psychiatric illness
C   more than two administration occasions per day
D   inconvenient clinics
E   family instability

1.21 **The following statements about prescription and administration of drugs in hospital are correct:**

A   The concept of compliance applies to patients but not to doctors
B   If doctors wrote cheques on their bank accounts as badly as they commonly write prescriptions they would soon be in trouble
C   Errors in drug administration in hospitals have been found to occur in about 20% of cases
D   Giving physicians information on drugs improves prescribing substantially
E   Asking physicians to justify their prescriptions has no effect except to annoy them

1.22 **Medicines in the home**

A   in most case are not doctor-prescribed
B   are found in about one house in ten
C   are usually kept in a locked cupboard or drawer, inaccessible to children
D   are most commonly kept in the bathroom
E   should be confined to those suitable for short-term relief of symptoms, such as pain, except where a medicine is in use according to medical direction

2 Clinical Pharmacology

2.1 Clinical pharmacology, the scientific study of drugs in man

A is a discipline called into existence by need

B comprises pharmacodynamics, pharmacokinetics, formal therapeutic trials and surveillance studies

C is so complex that it can only be conducted by specialist clinical pharmacologists

D raises problems that require experiments in animals for elucidation

E is fundamentally different from basic pharmacological science conducted on non-human animals or tissues

3 Discovery and Development of Drugs

3.1 In discovering and developing new drugs

A a principal approach is to synthesise agonist or antagonist analogues of naturally-occurring hormone or transmitter substances

B modification of structures of existing drugs cannot produce major differences

C knowledge of mode of action of a drug is not particularly useful for predicting effects in man from studies in animals

D induction of experimental diseases in animals (such as schizophrenia or depression), provides an ideal test system for studies predictive for man

E knowledge of kinetics of a drug in a test species allows toxicology tests to be designed with maximum relevance to use of the drug in man

3.2 In the development of new drugs

A differences in drug response between species, including man, are more commonly pharmacodynamic than pharmacokinetic

B a crude measure of safety of a drug may be obtained by dividing the plasma concentration providing therapeutic effect by the plasma concentration causing adverse effect

C toxicity tests in animals are generally confined to 6 months' duration (except for oncogenicity) even though the drugs may be used in man for years

D testing of all new drugs on pregnant animals has been mandatory since the thalidomide disaster

E national registers of birth defects, competently kept, plus accurate records of drug consumption should ensure that no major drug-induced defect in the fetus will be overlooked

3.3 **The following statements about mutagenesis and oncogenesis are correct:**

A Testing in animals for oncogenicity and mutagenicity should be mandatory for all new drugs, even those that are intended for short-term use, before they are given to man

B If a drug is mutagenic this effect will be detectable early during its administration

C Mutagens may also be carcinogens

D Drug-induced cancer may occur many years after the patient has stopped using the drug

E Cytotoxic anti-cancer drugs are also carcinogenic

3.4 **The following statements about special toxicology (reproduction, mutagenesis, carcinogenesis) are correct:**

A If a drug is teratogenic in an animal species it may not be used in women of reproductive age

B A positive laboratory mutagenicity test should bar the use of a substance in humans

C If the first generation offspring of a male human are normal then a mutagenic effect on his reproductive cells has not occurred

D Some drugs that are carcinogenic are in use in routine therapy

E If a drug is under suspicion for carcinogenicity a case control study is likely to be helpful

4 Evaluation of Drugs in Man: Therapeutic Trials

4.1 Rational introduction of a potential new drug comprises

A pharmacodynamic and pharmacokinetic studies on healthy subjects or patients

B use on patients to detect potential therapeutic utility

C formal controlled trials

D monitoring for adverse reactions (and efficacy) after release for general prescribing

E the submission of research studies in man to an ethics review committee

4.2 Regulatory guidelines for introduction of a new drug

A require evidence of bioavailability of a formulation

B do not require studies on interaction with other drugs

C state that at least one ingredient of a fixed-dose combination must be relevant to the patient's need

D require that a proprietary product be accompanied by a Data (information) Sheet

E ordinarily require at least three independent therapeutic trials to support a licence application for general use

4.3 The following statements about the evaluation in man of new drugs are correct:

A A new drug should only be tested in man if animal experiments predict a clear advantage

B All useful drug actions can be demonstrated in healthy volunteers

C Drug studies in man where there is no possibility of benefit to the subject are an accepted part of the process of developing new drugs

D Bioavailability and bioequivalence are the same thing

E Good practice requires that patients who have not completed a drug trial regimen be excluded from the final analysis

4.4 Formal therapeutic trials are particularly efficient at detecting

A rare adverse drug effects

B the efficacy of a drug in uncomplicated disease of mild to moderate severity

C effects in pregnant women

D unexpected therapeutic actions

E drug interactions

4.5 In the clinical evaluation of therapy the following statements are correct:

A Physicians who follow their judgement aided only by personal experience and intuition are not engaging in experiments

B A scientific experimental approach to therapeutics is inherently less ethical than practice guided by clinical experience and impression

C General impressions are never to be trusted

D Clinical impressions are always wrong

E If a patient gets better after treatment it is reasonable to conclude that the recovery is due to the treatment

4.6   Therapeutic trials are designed to show as far as is practicable

A   whether a treatment is of value
B   how great is its value
C   in what type of patients it is of value
D   what is the best method of applying the treatment
E   what are the disadvantages or dangers of a treatment

4.7   Features of the classic randomised controlled therapeutic trial include

A   precisely framed question to be answered
B   equivalent groups of patients
C   groups formed by allocating alternate patients to each treatment under investigation
D   treatments carried out concurrently
E   double-blind technique where evaluation depends on strictly objective measurements

4.8   Placebo or dummy medication

A   provides a control device by which true pharmacodynamic effects of therapy are distinguished from the general psychological effects of medication
B   provides a device to avoid false negative conclusions
C   is inherently unethical
D   is always scientifically necessary in a trial of drug therapy
E   is sometimes used in patients who also receive a pharmacologically active treatment

4.9 In a therapeutic trial

A   different treatments must never be given to the same patient
B   the order in which treatments are given may influence the results
C   the theoretical basis of the design is to test the hypothesis that there is no difference between the treatments under test
D   there is a risk of finding a difference where there is in reality no difference
E   there is no risk of finding no difference where there is in reality a difference

4.10 A statistical significance test

A   is a device concerned with probabilities rather than with certainties
B   when negative is of little interest unless the confidence interval is also stated and is narrow
C   plus a statement of confidence interval helps to avoid a Type 1 error
D   cannot be of use in cross-over studies
E   showing $P = 0.05$ means that if the experiment were repeated 100 times, there being in reality no difference between the treatments, then a difference as great as that observed would occur 5 times as a result of chance

4.11 A statistician

A   can salvage a poorly designed experiment after it has been completed
B   cannot tell the clinician how many patients he will need in a therapeutic trial to get a clinically important result unless the clinician can be explicit on the differences he expects and the risk he is prepared to accept of getting a misleading result (Type I error, Type II error)
C   contributes both to the precision of a therapeutic experiment and to its ethics
D   prefers sequential analysis reliably to detect small differences in multiple measurement, eg in arthritis
E   is likely to advise that a simple significance test conducted at regular intervals, the trial ceasing as soon as a positive result is obtained, is the best way of deciding when to stop a trial

4.12   Statistical principles and calculations

A   are invariably required to validate therapeutic efficacy
B   can prove that differences between treatments are clinically important
C   promote the making of wise decisions in the face of uncertainty
D   can validate therapeutic differences in data extracted from hospital case records
E   should be applied only where the design of the study is such that systematic biases in allocation of patients to treatment groups have been eliminated

4.13   The following statements about therapeutic trials are correct:

A   Knowledge of the results of a therapeutic trial conducted in groups of patients does not help the physician faced with an individual patient
B   A clinician who is personally convinced that treatment A is better than treatment B cannot ethically engage in a scientific study on the subject
C   Once a therapeutic trial has given a positive result it becomes unethical to do another similar trial
D   To conduct a scientific study in which the patient's treatment is chosen by random allocation is inherently unethical
E   A good guide to conduct is that no patient participating in a therapeutic trial should be worse off than he or she might otherwise have been in the hands of a competent doctor

4.14   A case control study

A   involves a retrospective approach and thus is inherently less valid scientifically than a prospective study such as the randomised controlled trial
B   reveals associations but does not prove causation
C   involves collecting a control group of subjects similar in essentials but without the condition under study
D   involves taking a drug history from each subject in order to compare the incidence of consumption (in each group) of the drug under suspicion (of an adverse effect)
E   gives results quicker than does an observational cohort study

5 Drug Regulation or Control

5.1 The following statements about official drug regulation and its history are correct:

A Modern comprehensive official drug regulation began in the USA (1938) after an accident involving sulphanilamide and diethylene glycol

B The company making the mixture tested it for fragrance and flavour but not for safety

C The lack of testing for safety did not infringe the then law in the USA

D The rest of the world only accepted the need for comprehensive control following the thalidomide disaster (1961)

E No new drug should be licenced for general prescribing (marketed) until it has been proved unable to do harm

5.2 Official drug regulation or control is concerned with

A quality of the manufactured drug and formulation

B safety of the drug

C efficacy of the drug

D supply to the medical profession and the public

E compiling a register of accepted medicinal products

5.3 A modern effective drug regulatory authority requires evidence of

A studies on animals

B chemical and pharmaceutical quality

C pharmacological studies in man

D formal therapeutic trials

E post licencing (marketing) surveillance

5.4 The following statements are correct:

A There are risks in taking drugs
B There are no risks in not taking drugs
C Introduction of a new drug into general use should be a gradual supervised process, not an abrupt one of licence or no licence
D The pursuit of 'safety at any cost' must be correct otherwise humans are unacceptably hazarded
E It is harder to detect and quantitate a *harm* that *is* done than it is to detect a *good* that is *not* done

5.5 Drug regulators

A should not take risks on behalf of society
B face uncertainty as to the true facts about a new drug at the time when they have to decide whether or not to grant a licence for general use
C are in the business of taking simple scientific decisions based on the evidence submitted to them
D are not prone to defensive practices
E could well have as a motto, "It seemed the right thing to do at the time"

5.6 The following statements about thalidomide are correct:

A Thalidomide injury was particularly in the children of professional social classes
B Thalidomide caused major anatomical abnormalities in fetuses when taken by the mother in the final six weeks of pregnancy
C Testing of new drugs for effects on reproduction may be confined to the period of organogenesis without losing capacity to predict risks to the fetus
D Thalidomide was recognised as harmful to fetuses as early as it was because it caused a very severe effect that was ordinarily seen extremely rarely
E When thalidomide was first suspected a case control study was quickly done

6 Classification of Drugs: Names of Drugs

6.1 The following statements are correct:

A Classification is a fundamental requirement of a science

B Nomenclature is a fundamental requirement of science

C A drug or medicine generally has three names

D Proprietary names apply to pure drug substances rather than to formulations

E There is a single classification of drugs that suits all interested parties

6.2 Drugs are generally classified by their

A proprietary names

B adverse effects

C mode of action

D chemical structure

E therapeutic use

6.3 The following statements about nomenclature of drugs are correct:

A Proprietary names are chosen to emphasise the similarities between similar drugs

B Official (non-proprietary) names are chosen to emphasise the differences between related drugs

C The full chemical name is best for prescribing purposes

D There is never a medically important reason for using a proprietary name in prescribing

E The majority of mixtures of drugs do not have non-proprietary names

7   How Drugs Act

7.1   The following statements about how drugs act are correct:

A   Living creatures, plants and animals, often produce toxic substances the effect of which is confined to their own genus

B   The heart of modern pharmacology is selective action between tissues

C   An inhibitor of enzyme-mediated synthesis is a substance that fits one active site of an enzyme but which is sufficiently unlike the usual substrate to fail to react with the substrate molecule fitted into the adjacent active site

D   An inhibitor of enzyme-mediated degradation is a substance that fits an active site of an enzyme so that the catalytic function of the enzyme is blocked and the natural substrate remains intact

E   When a molecule offered to an enzyme is so similar to its normal substrate that it can be used in synthetic reaction, the product may be biologically active, eg as a false transmitter

7.2 **The following statements about how drugs act are correct:**

A Drugs may alter the flow of ions across cell membranes

B Substances specially needed by cells may be subject to special active chemical pumping mechanisms

C Cells are provided with special macromolecular sites the conformation of which fits specific chemicals and which activate biological processes within the cell. These are called receptors

D There is only one type of receptor for each chemical transmitter or drug

E As concentration rises drugs become less selective (binding to low affinity sites) and unwanted effects increasingly appear

8 General Pharmacology

8.1 Drugs may act

A through enzyme inhibition
B by being incorporated into larger molecules
C outside the cell
D by chelation
E by osmotic effect

8.2 The following statements about drug action on cell membranes are correct:

A Antihistamines act on specific receptors
B Volatile anaesthetics act on specific receptors
C Cardiac antidysrhythmia drugs interfere with selective passage of ions
D Drugs may act through membrane-bound enzymes
E Drugs act on cell membrane constituents themselves

8.3 The following statements about drugs and receptors are correct:

A Agonists exert their principal effect by blockading receptors
B Antagonists exert their principal effect by activating receptors
C Naloxone is a pure antagonist
D Pindolol has partial agonist activity
E Phenoxybenzamine binds irreversibly to the α-adrenoceptor

8.4 Competitive antagonism

A   can be reversed by increasing the amount of agonist present

B   can be said to be present when the log-dose-response curve to agonist alone is not parallel to the curve obtained when an antagonist is present

C   is exemplified by the use of ethanol in methanol poisoning

D   never occurs with enzymes

E   is the same as physiological antagonism

8.5 The following drugs act principally by inhibiting enzymes:

A   Captopril

B   Carbidopa

C   Aspirin

D   Atropine in the management of overdose with a beta-blocker

E   Adrenaline in anaphylactic shock

8.6 The following statements about dose and response are correct:

A   Loop diuretics have a dose-response curve that reaches a maximum after a few increments of dose

B   Thiazide diuretics have a steep and prolonged dose-response curve

C   If one drug has greater therapeutic efficacy than another then it is more potent

D   If one drug is more potent than another drug then it can achieve a therapeutic effect of greater magnitude

E   The therapeutic index is the maximum tolerated dose divided by the minimum curative dose

8.7 **The following statements about the order of drug metabolic reaction processes are correct:**

A Processes for which rate is proportional to concentration are termed first order

B Processes for which the rate is constant regardless of changes in concentration are termed zero order

C First order processes exhibit saturation kinetics

D Alcohol in 'social' doses is metabolised by a zero order process

E Phenytoin is eliminated by first order processes throughout the clinical dose range

8.8 **First order processes**

A apply only to enzyme-mediated processes

B proceed at high rates when the concentrations of substances are high and vice versa

C can properly be described in terms of t½

D apply to most drugs in clinical use

E apply to salicylate metabolism throughout the therapeutic dose range

8.9 **In zero order kinetics**

A elimination rate is independent of dose

B the t½ is constant despite rising drug concentration

C enzyme mediated metabolic reactions become saturated

D uniform increases in dose may result in disproportionate increases in plasma concentration

E passive diffusion processes become saturated

8.10　**The following statements about drug t½ are correct:**

A　A drug of t½ 6 h that is present in the plasma at a steady concentration of 100 mg/l will have a concentration of 25 mg/l 18 h after administration is discontinued

B　A drug administered at 6 h intervals and having a t½ of 6 h will, after 12 h, attain a plasma concentration that is 75% of the ultimate steady state concentration

C　The time for a drug to reach steady state concentration in plasma is a function only of t½

D　When a drug is at steady state concentration in plasma and a different, regularly administered, dose is given, a new steady state concentration will be attained in two t½s

E　A drug that is given by repeated oral administration can be said to have reached steady state concentration in plasma when all peaks are of equal height

8.11　**The t½ of**

A　benzylpenicillin is 30 min
B　propranolol is 24 h
C　digoxin is 36 h
D　warfarin is 6 h
E　amiodarone is 700 h

8.12　**Drug plasma concentration is not worth measuring in the case of**

A　oral anticoagulants
B　diuretics
C　monoamine oxidase inhibitors
D　most antiepilepsy drugs
E　hypoglycaemics

8.13 **Factors that make it difficult to establish correlation between drug plasma concentration and pharmacological effect include**

A   the presence in the plasma of pharmacologically active metabolites
B   the use of an assay technique that measures pharmacologically inactive metabolites
C   the use of an assay technique that measures total (bound + free) drug in plasma
D   the presence of a 'therapeutic window'
E   the irreversible action of 'hit and run' drugs

8.14 **Monitoring of plasma concentration of drugs is a useful guide to therapy**

A   in some cardiac dysrhythmias
B   in drug overdose
C   with lithium
D   irrespective of the timing of blood sampling in relation to that of dosing
E   with diuretics

8.15 **Passage of drug across cell membranes**

A   by diffusion requires cellular energy
B   by diffusion exhibits first order kinetics
C   by filtration is most readily accomplished by neutral (uncharged) molecules
D   by filtration occurs at the renal glomerulus
E   by active transport may involve competition with other molecules of similar structure

8.16 **If the pH of a medium containing**

A a drug is the same as the pKa of the drug, then the drug is 50% ionised

B an acidic drug is increased by one unit, then the drug becomes 91% ionised

C a basic drug is decreased by two units, then the drug becomes 99% un-ionised

D aspirin (pKa 3.5) is 1.5, then the drug is 99% un-ionised

E pethidine (pKa 8.6) is 6.6, then the drug is 99% ionised

8.17 **The following statements about passage of drugs across cell membranes are correct:**

A Un-ionised drug is lipid soluble and diffusible

B The acidic environment of the stomach favours absorption of aspirin from that site

C Aspirin localises in the gastric epithelial cells (pH 7.4) by ion trapping

D Polar (permanently charged) drugs readily cross cell membranes

E Levodopa is actively transported across the blood brain barrier

8.18 **The following statements about drug ionisation are correct:**

A Acidic groups become less ionised in an acid medium

B The pKa is the negative logarithm of the Ka (ionisation constant)

C Two drugs having the same pKa will necessarily have the same lipid solubility

D pKa varies with environmental pH

E Many drugs are weak electrolytes

8.19 **The following statements about drug absorption from the gastrointestinal tract are correct:**

A The buccal route of administration gives rapid effect because it avoids first-pass inactivation in the liver

B The stomach is a major site of drug absorption

C The rate of gastric emptying can have a major influence on drug absorption

D Enterohepatic recycling helps to retain oral contraceptive steroids in the body

E The colon is incapable of absorbing drugs

8.20 **Bioavailability**

A refers to the amount of drug that is released from a dose form

B is highly dependent on the size of the particles of which a tablet is made

C is influenced by diluting substances within a dose form

D of different formulations is demonstrated by measuring plasma concentration-time profiles following administration of the same dose to individuals one after another

E differences may be the cause of unexpected drug toxicity or failure of therapy

8.21 **Pre-systemic elimination**

A may account for differences in enteral and parenteral drug dosages that achieve comparable effect

B is significant in the case of morphine administered by the oral route

C is significant in the case of chlormethiazole administered by the oral route

D is significant in the case of diazepam administered by the oral route

E may be reduced if the liver is diseased

8.22 Enteral administration

A of an antimicrobial drug should in general take place when the stomach is empty

B of gentamicin is the preferred route for systemic effect

C of solid dose forms should ideally take place lying down

D of a drug by the buccal route can be terminated rap dly

E of a drug by the rectal route may be advantageous in motion sickness

8.23 Rectal administration of drugs

A is particularly effective because absorption into the portal system and first pass elimination in the liver are largely avoided

B usually necessitates smaller doses than oral administration to achieve the same effect

C may be useful in migraine

D may cause proctitis

E is useful for drugs that irritate the stomach

8.24 Parenteral administration

A of a drug by the intravenous route may need to take account of the rate of blood circulation

B of oxytocin is the preferred route because its t½ is a few minutes

C of a drug by intramuscular injection in a patient with peripheral circulatory failure is accompanied by delayed absorption

D of a drug by inhalation is used only for local effect in the lung

E of a drug through the skin may give a reliable systemic effect

8.25   The apparent distribution volume

A   of a drug is the volume of fluid in which it appears to
      distribute with a concentration equal to that in plasma
B   of a drug is small if it remains in the plasma
C   of a drug normally corresponds precisely with a
      physiological space such as extracellular water
D   of a drug can not exceed total body volume
E   of warfarin is 8 l/kg in a 70 kg person

**8.26   On the basis of apparent volume of distribution,
          haemodialysis would be effective in removing drug from
          subjects overdosed with**

A   propranolol
B   pethidine
C   salicylate
D   digoxin
E   nortriptyline

**8.27   The following statements about drug binding to plasma
          proteins and tissues are correct:**

A   Bound drug is pharmacologically active
B   The main binding protein for many drugs in albumin
C   Drug protein binding may be reduced in chronic renal
      disease
D   Adverse reactions due to competition for protein binding
      are most likely with drugs having a large distribution
      volume
E   Quinidine and digoxin compete for binding sites in tissues

8.28   Drug distribution may be influenced by

A   body fluid pH
B   regional blood flow
C   plasma protein binding
D   lipid solubility
E   binding to body tissues for which they have strong affinity

8.29 Drug metabolism

A generally results in metabolites having increased lipid solubility

B generally converts a pharmacologically active to an inactive substance

C in the case of amitriptyline converts a pharmacologically active substance to another active substance

D in the case of enalapril converts a pharmacologically inactive substance to an active substance

E by conjugation normally terminates biological activity

8.30 Enzyme induction

A with antiepilepsy drugs may cause osteomalacia

B contributes to tolerance to the effects of alcohol

C enables the body to adapt to varying exposure to foreign compounds

D can affect plasma bilirubin concentration

E is usually brought about by lipid insoluble substances with short t½

8.31 Enzyme induction

A may be a cause of failure of oral contraceptive steroid

B may occur with a diet that includes barbecued meats and Brussels sprouts

C may be a cause of failure of anticoagulant control with warfarin

D caused by heavy alcohol consumption may be a cause of failure of expected drug response

E is not caused by tobacco smoke

8.32 Enzyme inhibition

A due to cimetidine reduces the effects of concurrently administered propranolol

B due to allopurinol is used in the treatment of alcoholism

C due to captopril is used in the treatment of hypertension

D due to monoamine oxidase inhibitors increases the effect of some sympathomimetics

E due to sodium valproate increases the effect of phenytoin

8.33 **The following statements about drugs in breast milk are correct:**

A As the pH of milk is more acidic than that of plasma basic drugs will accumulate in milk
B Binding to milk proteins is about half that to plasma proteins
C Some diuretics may suppress lactation before it is well established
D Use of aminophylline by a breast feeding mother may cause her infant to become irritable
E Repeated use of a benzodiazepine by a breast feeding mother may result in sedation of her infant

8.34 **The following statements about drug clearance are correct:**

A Renal clearance of a drug that is eliminated only by filtration by the kidney cannot exceed the glomerular filtration rate
B Total body clearance is usually given by the sum of the renal and hepatic clearances
C The renal clearance value of 480 ml/min for benzylpenicillin indicates that this drug is secreted by the renal tubules
D Substances having a molecular weight of 10,000 are excluded from the glomerular filtrate
E Passage into breast milk is an important route of drug elimination

8.35 **The following statements about drug dosing are correct:**

A For a drug with a t½ of >24 h, the daily maintenance should equal the amount of drug that leaves the body in 24 h
B For a drug with a t½ of <3 h, administering half the priming dose at intervals equal to the t½ is an acceptable regimen
C Drugs with long t½ are especially suitable for administration as sustained release preparations
D Combining a drug injected s.c. with adrenaline can be expected to shorten its duration of action
E Probenecid accelerates the excretion of penicillin

8.36   Fixed-dose drug combinations

A   are appropriate for the treatment of tuberculosis
B   are appropriate for the treatment of Parkinson's disease
C   are appropriate for drugs with a wide range of dose
D   facilitate the identification of adverse effects
E   may appropriately include adrenocortical steroids

8.37   Genetic variation

A   may explain lack of response to normal doses of warfarin
B   may be the cause of vitamin D resistant rickets
C   may be the cause of adverse reaction to hydralazine
D   in response to drugs exhibits discontinuous variation if monofactorial
E   may explain failure to breathe after a surgical operation

8.38   The following statements about age and drugs are correct:

A   Drugs are absorbed less readily through the skin of the infant than the adult
B   Distribution of drugs is influenced by the lower proportion of fat and the higher proportion of water in the neonate
C   Drug metabolism is especially slow in the neonate
D   Serum creatinine is a reliable indicator of the capacity to eliminate drugs by the kidney in the elderly
E   Drugs that act on the nervous system have reduced effect in the elderly

8.39   Pharmacokinetics may be influenced by

A   pregnancy
B   labour
C   partial gastrectomy
D   chronic liver disease
E   severe cardiac failure

8.40 Interaction between drugs

A with steep dose response curves is unlikely to be harmful
B with small therapeutic ratios is unlikely to be harmful
C is described as summation if the effects of two drugs having the same action are additive
D is described as potentiation if the action of one drug increases the effect of another
E may lead to valuable therapeutic effects

8.41 Addition of drugs to intravenous fluids

A will cause visible change in the solution if interaction occurs
B is safe in the case of heparin with penicillin
C is safe if the mixture is kept for several days before use
D is acceptable for blood, aminoacid solutions and fat emulsion
E may be rendered unsafe by the acidity of dextrose or sodium chloride solutions

8.42 Interactions of drugs in the gut may occur due to

A changes in pH
B changes in motility
C direct chemical reaction
D alteration of gut flora
E alteration of mucosal absorptive mechanisms

8.43 Drug interaction between

A naloxone and morphine occurs primarily at plasma protein binding sites
B unselective monoamine oxidase inhibitors and levodopa may lead to hypotension
C tricyclic antidepressants and antihypertensives may result in loss of antihypertensive effect
D rifampicin and warfarin may lead to increased anticoagulant effect
E phenytoin and the oral contraceptive pill may lead to pregnancy

8.44 **The following statements about clinically significant interactions resulting from enzyme inhibition by drugs are correct:**

A Drugs classed as monoamine oxidase (A+B) inhibitors alter clinical responses only to sympathomimetics
B Metronidazole and sulphonylureas alter clinical effects of alcohol
C Allopurinol inhibits azathioprine metabolism
D Chloramphenicol inhibits warfarin metabolism
E Isoniazid accelerates phenytoin metabolism

8.45 **Clinically important interactions between drugs**

A take place only in the body
B can occur only when drugs have the same site of action
C are invariably harmful
D may be antagonistic
E may be synergistic

9 Unwanted Effects of Drugs: Adverse Reactions

9.1 **The following statements about unwanted effects of drugs (adverse reactions) are correct:**

A There is a fundamental biological distinction between therapeutic and adverse effects of drugs

B Some adverse effects are due to normal predictable pharmacological effects of drugs and may occur in all patients taking the drug

C Some adverse effects are due to abnormalities in the patient and will only occur in some patients taking the drug

D The terms intolerant and tolerant refer to individuals at either extreme of the normal distribution curve

E Idiosyncrasy means allergy

9.2 **In evaluating adverse drug reactions as a source of disease it is useful to study their**

A nature

B severity

C incidence

D avoidability

E relationship to predisposing or causative factors in patients

9.3 In assessing the amount of disease that is caused by the practice of drug therapy the definition of an adverse drug reaction should include

A any unwanted effect, however small
B an effect that can be deemed actually harmful or seriously unpleasant
C accidental or deliberate overdose
D effects that warrant reduction of dose, withdrawal of the drug or foretell hazard from future administration
E avoidable as well as unavoidable effects

9.4 The following statements about adverse drug reaction detection are correct:

A Formal therapeutic trials reliably detect adverse reactions having an incidence of 1:10,000
B Spontaneous reporting systems provide reliable quantitative data on incidence of adverse reactions
C Drug-induced illness is often similar to spontaneous disease
D When monitoring new drugs recently licenced for general use doctors are asked to report all events, not only those they suspect to be due to the drug
E If it is desired reliably to detect a serious adverse reaction having an incidence of 1:10,000 (and no spontaneous incidence in the community) it will be necesary to monitor about 65,000 patients

9.5 In investigating the possibility of drug-induced illness the finding that

A a drug commonly induces an otherwise rare illness is detectable only with the utmost difficulty
B a drug rarely induces an otherwise common illness may go for ever undiscovered
C a drug rarely induces an otherwise rare illness is likely to be detected early in pre-licencing clinical trials
D a drug commonly induces an otherwise common illness is likely to be detected by informal clinical observation
E adverse reactions are a cause will be determined most reliably by clinical observation supported by case control and cohort studies

9.6 Adverse drug reactions

A cause 10% of consultations in general practice
B cause up to 3% of admissions to acute care hospital wards
C are particularly likely to occur in females over 60 years old
D are more likely to occur late rather than early in therapy
E are more likely to have a pharmacological rather than an immunological basis

9.7 Adverse drug reactions

A most commonly affect the cardiovascular and respiratory systems
B are uncommon in patients taking digoxin and diuretics
C often affect the gastrointestinal tract and skin
D do not follow the use of a placebo
E will not occur if a drug has been correctly chosen even if it is incorrectly used

9.8 Factors which may influence the incidence of adverse reactions to drugs include

A age
B sex
C genetic constitution
D disease
E tendency to allergy

9.9 Adverse drug reactions are influenced by

A inherent properties of the drug
B the choice of drug in a particular patient
C the way the drug is used
D the technique of manufacture of the pure drug
E other drugs the patients is taking

9.10 **The following statements about adverse drug reactions are correct:**

A Pharmacokinetic mechanisms are unimportant in causation

B Young children can be regarded as 'small adults' as far as liability to adverse drug reactions is concerned

C The first month of life is a period of special risk

D Old age is a period of special risk

E Older children metabolise some drugs more rapidly than do adults

9.11 **The elderly show an increased response to standard drug dosage and an increased incidence of adverse drug reactions because they have**

A increased lean body mass

B reduced renal and hepatic function

C reduced blood flow to vital organs

D better nutrition

E less efficient homeostatic mechanisms

9.12 **Patients having the following conditions tend to show a greater than normal response to many drugs:**

A Hypoalbuminaemia

B Congestive cardiac failure

C Hepatic cirrhosis

D Hyperthyroidism

E Hypothyroidism

9.13 **Hepatic porphyria**

A is an uncommon disease

B is due to a single gene defect

C may present as an acute illness after medication

D does not occur in patients treated with enzyme-inducing drugs

E may usefully be treated with fructose

9.14   **An attack of porphyria may be precipitated by**

A   aspirin
B   morphine
C   barbiturates
C   chlorpromazine
E   some 'home remedies', eg mouthwash

9.15   **The following statements are correct:**

A   Glaucoma in an asthmatic can safely be treated with
    β-adrenoceptor eye drops
B   A skin rash following use of ampicillin in a patient having a
    sore throat raises the possibility that the patient has
    porphyria
C   In peripheral circulatory failure from any cause drugs
    should not be injected subcutaneously
D   Hypopitutary patients are unusually tolerant of many
    drugs
E   In Hodgkin's lymphoma alcohol taken in social doses is
    liable to induce pain

9.16   **The following statements about drug allergy are correct:**

A   All drugs are antigens
B   If antibodies to a drug are present in patients, then they will
    suffer an adverse reaction if they receive the drug again
C   Drugs or drug metabolites combine with a body protein to
    form an antigen
D   Allergic reactions reproduce, only with greater intensity,
    the normal pharmacological actions of the causative drug
E   The chief target organs of drug allergy are skin, respiratory
    tract, gastrointestinal tract, blood, blood vessels

9.17 Where a drug causes an allergic (immunological) illness

A it is safe to change to another member of the same chemical class
B there is no linear relation of dose to effect
C safe desensitisation is impossible
D re-exposure to a small dose is enough to cause illness
E there has been a preceding first exposure followed by an interval

9.18 Important manifestations of drug allergy include

A thrombocytopenia
B granulocytopenia/agranulocytosis
C leukaemia
D aplastic anaemia
E haemolysis

9.19 Important manifestations of drug allergy include

A serum sickness syndrome
B asthma
C fever
D cholestatic jaundice
E collagen disease

9.20 In drug allergy

A laboratory tests are essential for diagnosis
B after recovery from a reaction, rechallenge with the suspected drug is both essential and safe
C skin tests give reliable diagnostic information for contact dermatitis only
D detection of drug-specific circulating antibodies is diagnostically conclusive that a suspected reaction was indeed allergic
E once allergy has occurred it is permanent

9.21 **Anaphylactic shock is an immunological condition in which**

A interaction of antigen with antibody causes cell damage with release of biologically active substances
B histamine is an important cause of the shock
C the blood pressure falls dramatically
D the bronchi dilate dramatically
E the emergency treatment is adrenaline given intramuscularly followed by a histamine H_1-receptor antagonist followed by an adrenocortical steroid

9.22 **Prevention of allergic reactions to drugs is assisted by**

A ensuring patients are clearly informed that they have an allergy
B paying attention to what patients tell you
C doing weekly blood counts on patients taking any drug known to produce blood disorders
D always taking a drug history from all patients
E desensitising (hyposensitising) all patients suspected of penicillin allergy

9.23 **In early pregnancy**

A drugs may damage the embryo or fetus indirectly by altering the mother's physiology
B the placenta readily allows water-soluble drugs to pass from mother to fetus
C once a drug enters the fetus it tends to persist longer than in the mother
D therapeutic effects on the fetus are sometimes achieved by giving drugs to the mother
E teratogens are likely to have their most devastating effects in early pregnancy

9.24 In late pregnancy or labour

A gross anatomical defects in the fetus are likely to result from drugs

B non-steroidal anti-inflammatory drugs can delay the onset of labour

C a vasoconstrictor drug given to the mother can cause fetal distress

D opioids given to the mother depress fetal respiration

E benzodiazepines given to the mother do not affect the fetus

9.25 Substances strongly suspected or known to be capable of harming the fetus when consumed by a pregnant woman include

A penicillin

B sex hormones

C antiepileptics

D warfarin

E alcohol

9.26 The following statements concerning teratogenicity are correct:

A The concept of absolute drug safety needs to be demolished

B In real life it can never be shown that a drug (or anything else) has no teratogenic activity at all

C When prescribing for a substantial period it is as important to consider whether a woman may become pregnant as whether she is already pregnant

D Some drugs in common use may be unrecognised low grade teratogens

E Fetal abnormality may be due to the disease for which the drug was prescribed

10 Drug Overdose, Poisoning and Antidotes

10.1 In self poisoning

A most cases represent an attempt to commit suicide
B domestic gas is still used as often as drugs
C there is a mortality rate of about 1% of acute hospital admissions
D the arthritic elderly are most likely to do it by accident
E benzodiazepines are among the drugs most often used

10.2 In acute poisoning

A the nature of the poison can be identified within a few hours by a Toxilab test
B naloxone antagonises opioid drugs
C gastric lavage should only be undertaken in children if they are conscious
D if it is decided to induce vomiting, saline solution is the safest medicine to give
E therapeutic emesis is contraindicated when a corrosive poison has been taken

10.3 In the treatment of acute poisoning

A by a central nervous system depressant it is more important to sustain the circulation than to wake the patient up
B gastric lavage is of no value more than 5 hours after a tricyclic antidepressant has been taken
C activated charcoal is ineffective in aspirin poisoning
D it is unlikely that more than 30% of the ingested drug will be recovered whatever measures are taken to empty the stomach
E gastric lavage is preferable to emesis if berries have been taken

10.4 In acute poisoning

A due to aspirin, simple infusion of sodium bicarbonate is at least as efficient as forced alkaline diuresis

B it is an advantage for a drug to be highly protein-bound when haemodialysis is undertaken

C peritoneal dialysis becomes inefficient in a hypotensive patient

D due to swallowing antifreeze solution haemodialysis is ineffective

E haemoperfusion may be unnecessary in theophylline poisoning if hypokalaemia is corrected

10.5 In the case of a patient unconscious due to drug overdose

A controlled ventilation may be needed to preserve oxygenation

B pulmonary oedema is a possible consequence of poisoning by β-adrenoceptor blockers

C an antimicrobial should be given to prevent hypostatic pneumonia

D if there is cardiac dysrhythmia, treatment with electrical pacing should be avoided

E resuscitation after cardiac arrest should be continued for longer than is customary

10.6 The following antidotes and their indications for use in poisoning are correctly paired:

A Calcium gluconate; indanedione anticoagulants

B Ethanol; methanol

C Phentolamine; β–adrenoceptor blocking agents

D Acetylcysteine; paracetamol

E Folinic acid: methotrexate

10.7 Dimercaprol

A acts by binding metal ions to its –SH groups
B may be life-saving in arsenic poisoning
C is only useful in lead poisoning if combined with sodium calciumedetate
D is given by deep intramuscular injection which causes pain
E causes hypertension

10.8 Penicillamine

A is more effective than dimercaprol in hepatolenticular degeneration (Wilson's disease)
B has to be given by injection
C has some beneficial effect in collagen disease
D causes no important adverse reaction
E has no effective substitute if it is not tolerated

10.9 In cyanide poisoning

A early symptoms are similar to those of anxiety
B there is irreversible chelation of the metallic part of cytochrome P_{450} oxidase
C specific treatment is by dicobalt edetate
D sodium thiosulphate is useful in the later stages of treatment
E treatment differs from that of carbon monoxide poisoning in that there is no place for hyperbaric oxygen

10.10 The following statements are correct:

A Sodium calciumedetate has revolutionised the treatment of lead poisoning
B Methanol overdose causes blindness that is transient, never permanent
C The breath of a patient with ethylene glycol poisoning has a characteristic smell
D The lungs are at great risk in poisoning with diesel oil
E Amanita phalloides is responsible for less than 50% of fatal 'mushroom' poisoning

10.11 **The following statements about herbicides and pesticides are correct:**

A Dinitro-orthocresol is not absorbed through the skin
B It is dangerous to use atropine to control sweating in poisoning by dinitro-compounds
C All rodenticides cause convulsions
D Paraquat is selectively taken up in the lungs
E Fuller's earth should be given urgently both in paraquat and in diquat poisoning

10.12 **CS, a common anti-riot agent**

A is a solid used in particulate aerosol form
B causes persistent bronchospasm even in normal people
C induces a transient rise in intra-ocular pressure
D has a plasma t½ of about 5 seconds
E causes excessive salivation which may persist for an hour

10.13 **Drugs which have probably been used for torture or 'interrogation' include**

A cyclophosphamide
B amphetamine
C thiopentone
D suxamethonium
E apomorphine

11 Infection I: Chemotherapy

11.1 The following drugs are primarily bactericidal

A sulphonamides
B tetracyclines
C aminoglycosides
D chloramphenicol
E rifampicin

11.2 The following statements about the mechanism of action of antimicrobial drugs are correct:

A Penicillin interferes with the peptidoglycan layer of the bacterial cell so that it absorbs water and bursts
B Amphotericin interferes with the cytoplasmic membrane of fungi
C Sulphonamides interfere with the build-up of peptide chains on ribosomes
D Tetracyclines prevent bacteria from synthesising folic acid
E Rifampicin interferes with bacterial nucleic acid metabolism

11.3 The choice of antimicrobial drugs

A may follow automatically from the clinical diagnosis if the causative organism is always the same and is always sensitive to the same drug
B should always be delayed until a positive identification of the infecting organism has been made
C should be based exclusively on *in vitro* sensitivity tests
D for pyogenic infections should only be altered after a trial of at least one week
E when bacteriological services are not available may best be a broad-spectrum combination

11.4   Combinations of antimicrobials are useful

A   to potentiate drug action, eg penicillin plus gentamicin for enterococcal endocarditis
B   to delay development of resistance, eg in tuberculosis
C   where treatment is essential before a diagnosis has been reached
D   to reduce the risk of suppression of normal flora
E   especially when a bactericidal drug is given with a bacteristatic drug

11.5   Chemoprophylaxis is justified

A   to prevent recurrent attacks of rheumatic fever
B   to prevent recurrence of acture glomerulonephritis
C   in epidemics of meningococcal meningitis
D   to prevent bacterial endocarditis after dental procedures
E   to prevent gas gangrene after mid-thigh amputation

11.6   Bacterial resistance to antimicrobials can arise

A   when naturally sensitive strains are eliminated, allowing naturally resistant organisms to proliferate
B   from spontaneous mutation
C   when sexual intercourse between cells allows the passage of plasmids
D   by passage of bacteriophage from one cell to another
E   through drug destroying enzymes produced by bacteria

11.7   Adverse consequences of antimicrobial drug use may include

A   opportunistic infections by *Clostridium difficile* causing colitis
B   opportunistic infection with *Candida albicans*
C   masking of infection, eg syphilis
D   inhibition of alcohol metabolism
E   ototoxicity

12 Infection II: Antibacterial Drugs

12.1 Penicillins

A are effective only against multiplying organisms
B are eliminated from the body only by glomerular filtration
C in all forms are resistant to degradation by gastric acid
D are presented as their sodium or potassium salts which may be significant in patients with cardiac or renal disease
E of the aminopenicillin type, eg amoxycillin, are indicated for infectious mononucleosis

12.2 Allergic reaction to penicillin

A may take the form of anaphylactic shock which can be fatal
B in an individual indicates that a cephalosporin may safely be given
C can be relied on to disappear spontaneously with passage of time
D in healthy people should always be managed by an attempt at hyposensitisation
E may be predicted by testing for specific IgE antibodies in the patient's plasma

12.3 Benzylpenicillin given alone is highly active against

A *Streptococcus pneumoniae* (pneumococcus)
B *Streptococcus pyogenes* (beta-haemolytic streptococcus)
C *Staphylococcus pyogenes* (beta-lactamase producing)
D *Neisseria meningitidis* (meningococcus)
E *Streptococcus faecalis* causing endocarditis

12.4   The following statements about penicillins are correct:

A   Ampicillin and amoxycillin are destroyed by beta-lactamase
B   Flucloxacillin and cloxacillin are resistant to beta-lactamase
C   Ticarcillin is particularly effective against *Pseudomonas aeruginosa*
D   Talampicillin is a prodrug for ampicillin
E   Piperacillin is inactive against *Pseudomonas aeruginosa*

12.5   Cephalosporins

A   do not have the beta-lactam ring in their structure
B   as a rule are excreted unchanged by the kidney
C   should not be used in patients who have had severe or immediate type allergic reactions to penicillin
D   in general have plasma t½s of less than 3 h
E   may cause thrombocytopenia and neutropenia if administration is continued for longer than 2 weeks

12.6   Aminoglycosides

A   are in general inactivated by metabolism in the liver
B   are in general active against aerobic Gram-negative organisms
C   are unsuitable to use in regimens to sterilise the bowel
D   may cause nephrotoxicity
E   such as neomycin used topically may be absorbed sufficiently to cause ototoxicity

12.7   Sulphonamides

A   act by preventing bacterial synthesis of folic acid
B   are more active after metabolism to the acetylated form
C   are more active in alkaline urine
D   may cause crystalluria
E   may cause the Stevens-Johnson syndrome

12.8 Co-trimoxazole

A is the treatment of choice for pneumonia due to *Pneumocystis carinii*
B is an alternative to chloramphenicol for enteric fever
C is being replaced by trimethoprim alone for urinary tract infections due to *E. coli*
D is being replaced by trimethoprim alone for respiratory tract infections due to *Haemophilus influenzae*
E is a combination of trimethoprin and clavulanic acid

12.9 A member of the tetracycline class of antibiotic

A is better absorbed from the intestinal tract if taken with dairy products
B is as a rule excreted unchanged in the urine
C such as demeclocycline may be used to treat hyponatraemia due to the syndrome of inappropriate antidiuretic hormone secretion
D is effective against *Mycoplasma pneumoniae* infection
E is the treatment of choice for chlamydial salpingitis

12.10 Tetracyclines can cause

A liver damage, especially in pregnancy
B decreased sensitivity to dental caries
C photosensitisation
D opportunistic infection with yeasts and moulds
E serious growth retardation in children treated for chronic respiratory disease

12.11 The following statements about antimicrobial drugs are correct:

A Erythromycin is the drug of choice for Legionnaires' disease
B Erythromycin estolate can cause cholestatic hepatitis
C Metronidazole is effective for trichomoniasis of the urogenital tract
D Metronidazole is ineffective for infection with anaerobic organisms
E Metronidazole accelerates the metabolism of alcohol

12.12 **The following statements about antimicrobial drugs are correct:**

A   Chloramphenicol is inactivated slowly by the neonate
B   Chloramphenicol is effective treatment for infection with *Haemophilus influenzae*
C   Aplastic anaemia due to chloramphenicol may be either an allergy or a dose-related response
D   Clindamycin penetrates bone and joints well
E   Sodium fusidate is effective treatment for infection with beta-lactamase-producing staphylococci

12.13 **The following statements about antimicrobial drugs are correct:**

A   Spectinomycin is used for gonorrhoea in patients allergic to penicillin
B   Acrosoxacin is effective treatment for syphilis
C   Vancomycin plus an aminoglycoside is effective treatment for streptococcal endocarditis in patients who are allergic to benzylpenicillin
D   Vancomycin is effective in pseudomembranous colitis due to *Clostridium difficile*
E   Mupirocin is much more effective in the treatment of folliculitis and impetigo if given systemically rather than topically

13 Infection III: Chemotherapy of Bacterial Infections

13.1 In a case of septicaemia

A treatment is so urgent that it should be started before taking blood cultures

B *Streptococcus pneumoniae* is a more likely pathogen than streptococcus Group B in the newborn

C *Staphylococcus aureus* is a likely cause in all age groups

D antimicrobials should be given parenterally

E with hypotension due to toxins, Gram-negative organisms are always responsible

13.2 The following statements are correct:

A *Haemophilus influenzae* is not a likely cause of infection of the auditory canal in children

B Middle ear infection may be caused by *mycobacterium tuberculosis*

C In sinusitis, antimicrobials have dispensed with the need to promote normal drainage

D A bulging inflamed eardrum demands treatment by myringotomy

E In sinusitis it is easy to decide what organism is responsible once cultures have been made

13.3 In throat infections

A chemotherapy is not of great importance unless streptococci have been cultured

B benzylpenicillin should be given in even a mild case of scarlet fever

C chemoprophylaxis should be continued for life after a second attack of rheumatic fever

D Vincent's infection demands treatment with metronidazole as benzylpenicillin is now ineffective

E due to diphtheria, there is no longer any need for antitoxin, provided that erythromycin is used

13.4 In the treatment of bronchitis

A acute infection responds well to amoxycillin

B suppressive chemotherapy for chronic infection is generally needed only during the colder months

C years of chemotherapy may be avoided by giving up smoking

D with airways obstruction, corticosteroids are as effective as they are in asthma

E there is no place for the use of disodium cromoglycate

13.5 The following statements about pneumonia are correct:

A A cephalosporin is preferable to benzylpenicillin for all patients with lobar pneumonia

B Atypical pneumonia due to *Mycoplasma pneumoniae* is treated by erythromycin

C *Klebsiella pneumoniae* infection in an elderly debilitated patient is treated by cefuroxime plus an aminoglycoside

D *Pneumocystis carinii* pneumonia in a patient suffering from AIDS is treated by co-trimoxazole

E Legionnaires' disease responds to benzylpenicillin

13.6　In infective endocarditis

A　treatment should not be delayed once blood cultures have been taken, even if the organism has not been identified

B　enterococci are isolated more often in older than in younger patients

C　with proper techniques the causal organism can be isolated in over 95% of cases

D　more prolonged therapy is required in patients with infected prosthetic valves

E　a fungal cause may go unrecognised for months after cardiac surgery

13.7　With regard to the prophylaxis of infective endocarditis in patients who are at risk

A　an antimicrobial should be administered for two days prior to a dental or surgical procedure

B　patients with prosthetic heart valves should not be anaesthetised outside hospital for dental procedures

C　antibiotic cover is obligatory for fibreoptic endoscopy

D　prophylactic antibiotics are not required for genitourinary procedures unless the urine is infected

E　patients undergoing tonsillectomy who are allergic to penicillin require intravenous vancomycin and gentamicin

13.8　In meningitis

A　a history of middle ear infection favours a pneumococcal aetiology

B　due to *Haemophilus influenzae* the patient is likely to respond to benzylpenicillin

C　of meningococcal origin patients allergic to penicillin should be treated initially with chloramphenicol

D　intrathecal treatment is life-saving in many cases

E　due to tuberculosis, isoniazid is of little value because of its failure to penetrate well into the CSF

13.9 **The following statements about intestinal infections are correct:**

A Treatment of typhoid fever with chloramphenicol prevents the development of a carrier state

B Even quite mild shigellosis demands treatment with co-trimoxazole

C *Campylobacter jejuni* is a leading cause of enteritis

D In cholera the most important aim of treatment remains rehydration and the maintenance of fluid balance

E Enteritis due to *Yersinia enterocolitica* carries a high mortality

13.10 **It is advantageous to suppress bowl flora in**

A hepatic insufficiency

B blind loop syndrome

C patients requiring intensive anti-leukaemia therapy

D ulcerative colitis

E patients being prepared for colonic surgery

13.11 **In the treatment of urinary tract infections**

A gentamicin is preferred to amoxycillin for asymptomatic infection in pregnancy

B recurrent infections are not diminished by chemoprophylaxis

C nitrofurantoin is a suitable drug for acute pyelonephritris

D nalidixic acid is active against *Proteus* spp

E quinolones such as ciprofloxacin may prove useful against Gram-negative organisms

13.12 In the treatment of infections of the genital tract

A *Treponema pallidum* never becomes resistant to penicillin
B the use of tetracyclines to treat gonorrhoea limits the incidence of co-existent chlamydia infection
C both non-specific vaginitis and trichomonas vaginitis respond well to metronidazole
D non-specific urethritis (NSU) does not respond to tetracycline
E the cure rate in syphilis treated with penicillin is as good in seropositive as in seronegative cases

13.13 In eye infections

A superficial infections are best treated with sulphacetamide drops
B acyclovir as an ointment is useful in herpes simplex keratitis
C due to a virus hydrocortisone may make the condition worse
D neomycin is nearly always effective in chlamydial conjunctivitis of the newborn
E oral tetracycline is effective in trachoma in developing countries whatever the serotype

13.14 The following statements about anti-tuberculosis treatment are correct:

A A combination of isoniazid and rifampicin is the cornerstone of short course continuous chemotherapy
B Non-compliance is the chief reason for failure of chemotherapy
C The chances of success of once-weekly regimes incorporating isoniazid are greater with slow acetylators
D Tuberculosis of the skin usually resists chemotherapy
E Adrenal steroids have a useful role in the treatment of severely ill patients

13.15 Isoniazid

A has little or no activity against bacteria other than
   Mycobacterium tuberculosis
B acts as efficiently in fast acetylators as in slow acetylators if
   given daily without other drugs
C has no effect on hepatic function
D is less likely to cause peripheral neuropathy if pyridoxine is
   also given
E may precipitate epilepsy

13.16 Rifampicin

A has a bactericidal action against tubercle bacilli
B is effective in leprosy
C should be discontinued and never used again if
   thrombocytopenia develops
D does not interfere with the efficacy of oral contraceptives
E causes an orange discolouration in soft contact lenses

13.17 Adverse effects of

A ethambutol include monocular retrobulbar neuritis
B pyrazinamide include arthralgia associated with a raised
   plasma uric acid
C aminosalicylic acid are both common and serious
D thiacetazone are likely to occur in patients with either
   hepatic or renal damage
E all antituberculosis drugs can be avoided by giving them in
   combination

13.18 Benzylpenicillin is the initial treatment of choice for

A leprosy
B gas gangrene
C osteomyelitis
D brucellosis
E leptospirosis

14 Infection IV: Chemotherapy of Viral, Fungal, Protozoal and Helmintic Infections

14.1 Acyclovir

A is a prodrug
B selectively inhibits viral DNA synthesis
C is effective by mouth and intravenously
D benefits herpes virus infections
E has remarkably few adverse effects

14.2 In the chemotherapy of viral infections

A idoxuridine should only be used topically in herpes infections
B vidarabine is especially useful in patients with encephalitis
C amantidine is effective in both influenza A and influenza B
D interferon is obtained from human cells in culture infected with a parainfluenza virus
E interferon is of no value in immunocompromised patients

14.3 In the chemotherapy of fungal infections

A nystatin is well absorbed from the alimentary tract
B amphotericin remains the drug of choice for most systemic infections
C ketoconazole is mostly used for superficial mycoses
D serious adverse effects have caused griseofulvin to be abandoned
E flucytosine is the most effective treatment for vaginal candidiasis

14.4 **The following statements about the treatment of an acute attack of malaria are correct:**

A Quinine no longer has a significant role to play
B Chloroquine is a drug of choice
C Fixed-dose combinations have no role
D Dexamethasone benefits cerebral malaria
E Antifols such as pyrimethamine are potentiated by sulphonamide derivatives such as dapsone

14.5 **The following statements about the prevention of malaria by drugs in a non-immune visitor to an endemic area are correct:**

A Preventive efficacy depends on starting to take the drug two weeks before exposure to infection
B Preventive efficacy depends on continuing the drug for six weeks after leaving the endemic area
C Primaquine eliminates the plasmodia from the body
D Chloroquine suppresses acute attacks without eliminating the plasmodia from the body
E Drug resistance of plasmodia is not a significant problem

14.6 **In amoebiasis**

A metronidazole is the agent of first choice for symptomatic tissue-invading disease
B emetine is no longer thought to damage the myocardium
C diloxanide is useful only in eradicating the cystic forms from the bowel lumen
D tetracycline has a part to play in the treatment of severe cases with extensive ulceration
E chloroquine is effective solely in hepatic amoebiasis

14.7 The following statements are correct:

A Suramin is particularly useful in the treatment of African trypanosomiasis with CNS involvement

B Chronic infection with *Giardia lamblia* responds to metronidazole

C If mebendazole is used for enterobiasis, it is not necessary to treat all members of the family

D There is no effective treatment for toxoplasmosis

E Diethylcarbamazine is used to treat filariasis

15 Inflammation and Non-steroidal Anti-inflammatory Drugs: Arthritis

15.1 Non-steroidal anti-inflammatory drugs

A cause sodium retention and oedema
B may be used to attempt closure of a patent ductus arteriosus
C reduce fever
D can cause asthma
E can protect against vascular occlusion

15.2 Paracetamol when taken in acute overdose

A characteristically causes immediate symptoms
B is rendered non-toxic by infusion of glutathione
C may be rendered non-toxic by acetylcysteine i.v.
D may cause serious liver and kidney damage
E may be effectively eliminated from the body by urine alkalinisation

15.3 The following statements about non-steroidal anti-inflammatory drugs are correct:

A Ibuprofen displaces coumarin anticoagulants from plasma protein binding sites, causing a clinically serious interaction
B Mefenamic acid may cause non-oliguric renal failure in the elderly
C Indomethacin may cause headache
D Sulindac is a prodrug
E Taken in combination over years they may impair renal function

15.4 **The following statements about aspirin and salicylates are correct:**

A Aspirin has a t½ of 5 h
B Salicylate has a t½ of 15 min
C Aspirin is more toxic to the stomach if taken with sodium bicarbonate
D Aspirin toxicity to the gut can be reduced by manipulating the formulation
E Aspirin reduces blood platelet adhesiveness

15.5 **Salicylates, including aspirin,**

A cause respiratory alkalosis in acute overdose
B in high dose shorten prothrombin time
C are metabolised according to zero-order kinetics at high therapeutic doses
D cause urate retention in ordinary therapeutic dose
E cause tinnitus in overdose

15.6 **Aspirin**

A causes gastrointestinal symptoms in about 1 in 15 of the population
B when taken with alcohol has a less risk of causing gastrointestinal haemorrhage than has aspirin on its own
C may cause gastrointestinal haemorrhage after a single dose
D when enteric-coated, causes less gastrointestinal bleeding
E when taken regularly causes loss of about 5 ml of blood per day from the gastrointestinal tract in most people

15.7 **Aspirin poisoning**

A is benefited by urinary acidification
B does not occur if enteric-coated formulations are used
C may cause severe metabolic acidosis especially in children under 4 years
D should be regarded as severe if the plasma salicylate exceeds 750 mg/l
E may require treatment with haemodialysis

15.8   In the treatment of rheumatoid arthritis

A   a propionic acid derivative is a reasonable first choice for mild disease

B   regular measurements of plasma salicylate are mandatory if aspirin is used

C   gold or penicillamine are most effective in preventing progression of the disease in early cases

D   adverse effects of gold may be treated with dimercaprol

E   penicillamine causes few adverse effects

15.9   In the treatment of rheumatoid arthritis

A   chloroquine gives benefit within 4 days

B   the therapeutic efficacy of sulphasalazine appears to equal that of gold

C   azathioprine has a useful corticosteroid-sparing effect

D   prednisolone may slow down aggressive or rapidly progressive disease

E   intra-articular injections of corticosteroid into a single joint should not exceed 2 or 3 per year

15.10   The following statements about hyperuricaemia and gout are correct:

A   Patients with gouty tophi have a urate pool that is 15–26 times normal

B   Hyperuricaemia may result from treatment of a myeloproliferative disorder

C   Colchicine relieves pain and inflammation of gout in a few hours

D   Probenecid is a useful analgesic for gout

E   Allopurinol is used in gout for its uricosuric action

15.11 In the treatment of gout

A initial use of sulphinpyrazone should be accompanied by a high fluid intake and alkalinisation of the urine
B indomethacin is a sound first choice for the acute condition
C allopurinol will provide useful relief from an acute attack
D a salicylate should be combined with a uricosuric
E a diuretic may cause relapse

16 Central Nervous System I: Pain and Analgesics: Drugs in Terminal Illness

16.1 The following statements about pain and analgesics are correct:

A Pain is the commonest symptom that takes a patient to a doctor
B Pain is defined as an unpleasant sensory, but not emotional, experience that occurs only in association with actual tissue damage
C All drugs that relieve pain should be classed as analgesics
D Only narcotic drugs can truly be called analgesics
E Non-analgesic, eg psychotropic, drugs can be useful adjuvants alongside analgesics

16.2 Pain is a complex phenomenon composed of a variable mix of

A nociceptive input
B input from other receptors
C anxiety, fear
D depression
E synthesis and release of local tissue hormones, eg prostaglandins, which cause inflammation and sensitise nerve endings that mediate pain

16.3 The following statements about pain are correct:

A Pain is a consequence of the activation of specific pain receptors in the affected tissue
B Acute and chronic pain are treated similarly
C Tissue injury always gives rise to pain
D Anxiety can intensify pain
E Depression makes a major contribution to 'suffering'

16.4 The following statements about pain are correct:

A There is a 'pain centre' in the brain
B There are natural endogenous opioid receptors in the central nervous system and these respond to administered opioids
C Naloxone competitively opposes administered opioids
D Naloxone does not cause spontaneous pain, but can make existing pain worse
E Non-steroidal anti-inflammatory drugs benefit pain by preventing prostaglandin synthesis

16.5 The following statements about acute and chronic pain are correct:

A In acute pain, once effective analgesia has been achieved, subsequent doses should be given to prevent recurrence
B In chronic pain adjuvant drugs are particularly useful
C In chronic pain it is best to inject analgesics
D In acute pain an analgesic with sedative action is unacceptable
E Tolerance to placebo effect does not occur

16.6 The following statements about testing of analgesic drugs are correct:

A Placebos give relief in about 35% of cases
B Emotional response to pain can largely be ignored in healthy volunteer experiments
C Double-blind technique is unnecessary
D Animal experiments are valueless
E The sex of the observer may affect the response of the patient to analgesics

16.7 The following statements about the choice of analgesics are correct:

A Analgesia for mild pain is best provided by paracetamol or aspirin

B Analgesia for moderate pain is best provided by a low-efficacy opioid combined if necessary with a non-steroidal anti-inflammatory drug

C Severe pain requires a high efficacy opioid combined with a low-efficacy opioid

D Overwhelming acute pain responds to a high-efficacy opioid plus a psychotropic drug, eg chlorpromazine

E The inclusion of caffeine in fixed-ratio analgesic combinations has no scientific basis

16.8 Pain

A from visceral smooth muscle responds best to aspirin

B from spasm of striated muscle should first be treated with an opioid

C of thalamic origin may respond to chlorpromazine

D of trigeminal neuralgia should in the first instance be treated with pentazocine

E of inflammation responds to aspirin

16.9 In a migraine attack

A vasoactive amines in the diet may play a causative role

B release of vasoactive amine from blood platelets may play a causative role

C the aura is due to cerebral vasodilation

D the pain is due to extracerebral vasoconstriction

E 90% of cases respond to early treatment with an appropriate mix of drugs

16.10 Drugs that are useful in an acute attack of migraine include

A paracetamol
B metoclopramide
C a benzodiazepine
D pethidine
E cyclizine

16.11 Ergotamine

A is valuable for preventing migraine
B in overdose can cause gangrene of the extremities by its α-adrenoceptor agonist action
C is safe to use in pregnancy
D is best avoided in obliterative vascular disease
E is needed in about 10% of acute attacks of migraine

16.12 Drugs that may be useful in prevention of recurrent migraine include

A aspirin
B propranolol
C verapamil
D pizotifen
E clonidine

16.13 The following statements regarding care of the terminally ill are correct:

A Symptom control is all-important to provide optimal quality of life
B Drugs play only a minor role in symptom control
C Morphine does not give useful analgesic effect when taken orally
D Tricyclic antidepressants have a morphine-sparing effect
E It is not acceptable practice to leave a dose of an opioid accessible to patients at night to be taken if they choose

16.14 In the patient terminally ill with cancer

A nerve compression may be relieved by prednisolone
B headache due to raised intracranial pressure responds to dexamethasone
C anorexia may be helped by prednisolone
D prostaglandin synthetase inhibitors are effective for bone pain due to metastases
E and in continuous pain the interval between doses of analgesics should be short enough to prevent pain recurring

16.15 Endorphins

A are naturally-occurring peptides
B counteract the analgesic activity of morphine
C are all short acting
D are not neurotransmitters
E probably play a part in the phenomena of opioid dependence and withdrawal

16.16 Morphine

A stimulates some functions of the central nervous system
B depresses some functions of the central nervous system
C tranquillises
D produces euphoria
E produces dysphoria

16.17 Morphine can cause

A diarrhoea
B vomiting
C biliary tract spasm
D antidiuresis
E miosis

16.18 Morphine should if possible be avoided in patients with

A pancreatitis
B asthma
C respiratory depression
D acute left ventricular failure
E ureteric colic

16.19 Morphine may safely be given

A subcutaneously to shocked patients
B to patients with hepatic failure
C to control diarrhoea
D together with a monoamine oxidase inhibitor
E repeatedly to patients with trigeminal neuralgia

16.20 Morphine and heroin dependence

A are more disabling socially and physically than is opium dependence
B should be treated by abrupt withdrawal of the drug
C are acceptable in the management of chronic pain in the terminally ill
D can occur within 24 hours if the drug is given 4-hourly
E can occur in infants born to addicted mothers

16.21 Codeine

A is as effective an analgesic as morphine
B does not constipate
C is a useful antitussive
D is widely used in fixed-ratio combinations
E is partly metabolised into morphine in the body

16.22 Pethidine

A has higher therapeutic efficacy than does morphine
B is preferred above codeine for cough suppression
C constipates
D is used in labour in preference to morphine
E has strong hypnotic effect

16.23 Methadone

A has a t½ much longer than that of morphine and pethidine
B dependence is less severe than is morphine dependence
C is widely used (orally) to help wean addicts from injected heroin
D blocks the acute effects of injected heroin
E is useful for severe cough

16.24 Heroin (diamorphine)

A has greater efficacy with less adverse effects than does morphine
B has only one proved advantage over morphine, ie that it is much more soluble
C has a plasma t½ of 3 minutes
D is metabolised in the body to morphine and to 6-acetylmorphine
E is used for very severe cough

16.25 The following statements about opioids are correct:

A Pentazocine and buprenorphine have both agonist and antagonist opioid activity
B Pentazocine may induce a withdrawal syndrome in opioid (heroin, morphine) dependent subjects
C Partial agonist opioids are free from the classic opioid adverse effects
D Neither pentazocine nor buprenorphine induce dependence
E Dihydrocodeine may make postsurgical dental pain worse

16.26 Naloxone

A is a non-competitive opioid antagonist
B is effective treatment for opioid overdose
C is longer acting than is morphine
D only partially antagonises buprenorphine
E does not induce an acute withdrawal syndrome in heroin addicts

17 Central Nervous System II: Sleep and Hypnotics: Anxiety and Anxiolytic Sedatives

17.1   A substance which

A   induces drowsiness, sleep or stupor especially with analgesia is called a *narcotic*

B   induces sleep is called a *hypnotic*

C   calms and soothes without inducing sleep is called a *sedative*

D   allays anxiety without materially impairing consciousness is called a *tranquillizer*

E   has antipsychotic effect may be called a *neuroleptic*

17.2   The following statements about sleep are correct:

A   Normal sleep is of two kinds

B   The kinds of sleep may be characterised by eye movement patterns or electroencephalographic patterns

C   Hypnotic-induced sleep is indistinguishable from normal sleep

D   Normal sleep patterns are resumed immediately on withdrawal of a hypnotic after a period of continuous use

E   All hypnotics can induce dependence

17.3   The following statements about hypnotics are correct:

A   If a patient does not feel a hangover after a hypnotic he can count on his psychomotor performance being normal

B   Hypnotics are best taken one hour before going to bed

C   After a long period of continuous use a hypnotic should be withdrawn slowly over weeks

D   Where a patient objects to withdrawal so strongly that it is impracticable a benzodiazepine is the hypnotic of choice

E   Barbiturates are never a first choice as a hypnotic

17.4 In treating insomnia

A prescription of a hypnotic is not justified to help a patient through a sudden distressing situation, e.g., bereavement, as it is just this sort of use that carries risk of dependence

B prescription of a hypnotic is the first choice if the insomnia is chronic

C it is important to make a detailed enquiry into its cause and pattern

D it should be remembered that sleep requirement becomes less with increasing age

E benzodiazepines are the first choice as hypnotics

17.5 The following statements about anxiety are correct:

A Anxiety is always harmful

B Anxiety does not always have an environmental or life-situational cause

C Non-drug therapy is a waste of time

D Surgeons who experience heart rates above 130/min in the operating theatre should take a pre-operative β-adrenoceptor blocker

E Long-term use of a benzodiazepine is desirable to ensure there is no relapse of anxiety

17.6 In the treatment of anxiety

A psychic symptoms respond particularly well to β-adrenoceptor blocking drugs

B somatic symptoms should be treated with an α-adrenoceptor blocking drug

C benzodiazepines are first choice drugs in acute cases

D benzodiazepines with a short t½ are preferred in chronic cases

E pre-examination panic in students cannot be benefited by drugs

17.7 Benzodiazepines

A are overprescribed for unhappiness
B only rarely induce dependence
C are without efficacy in epilepsy
D in overdose are particularly liable to cause respiratory depression
E can cause paradoxical excitement and aggression

17.8 Benzodiazepines

A reduce the activity of a central neurotransmitter, GABA (gamma-aminobutyric acid)
B cause anterograde amnesia
C are used as sedatives for endoscopy
D do not sedate sufficiently to render car driving inadvisable
E given to a mother in labour may depress suckling in the newborn infant

17.9 Benzodiazepines

A alter sleep pattern more than do other hypnotics
B are potent inducers of hepatic drug metabolising enzymes
C are safer if taken in overdose than are other hypnotics
D all have pharmacologically active metabolites
E having a long t½ are best for repeated use in insomnia

17.10 The following statements about hypnotics and sedatives are correct:

A Paraldehyde, subjected to light and heat, decomposes to acetic acid
B Paraldehyde dissolves plastic syringes
C Chloral hydrate is a prodrug
D Bromides still have a place in the treatment of nymphomania and spermatorrhoea
E Chlormethiazole is a hypnotic and sedative particularly advocated in alcoholism and the aged

17.11 Barbiturates

A have a low therapeutic index

B are all more easily eliminated with the aid of alkaline diuresis

C are potent inducers of hepatic drug metabolising enzymes

D cause only mild physical dependence

E are used for anaesthesia and convulsive states

18 Central Nervous System III: Drugs and Mental Disorder: Psychotropic or Psychoactive Drugs

18.1 Psychotropic drugs

A act by modifying chemotransmitter systems in the nervous system

B are more likely to be effective in neuroses than in psychoses

C act in the reticular activating system which particularly influences arousal

D act in the limbic system which particularly influences affect or emotion

E act in the hypothalamus which particularly influences the autonomic system

18.2 Schizophrenic states

A are particularly associated with dopaminergic activity in the brain

B are benefited by drugs that block dopamine receptors

C are benefited by the phenothiazine group of neuroleptics

D manifesting themselves with negative symptoms, eg apathy, respond particularly well to drug therapy

E manifesting themselves with positive symptoms, eg delusions, respond particularly poorly to drug therapy

18.3   Depressive states

A   are particularly associated with cholinergic activity in the brain
B   are benefited by drugs that block adrenoceptors in the brain
C   respond to drugs after 7–14 days
D   respond to electroconvulsive therapy even more slowly than to drugs
E   are currently best explained by changes in monoamine function in the brain

18.4   The following statements about mania and manic depressive disorder are correct:

A   Mania may be accompanied by overactivity of catecholamine transmission in the brain
B   Lithium may benefit mania by altering amine metabolism or receptor function
C   Lithium should only be used in severe cases of acute mania
D   A phenothiazine neuroleptic is a drug of first choice for acute mania
E   A butyrophenone neuroleptic is a drug of first choice

18.5   The following statements about the management of depression are correct:

A   For prevention of unipolar depression lithium is better than a tricyclic antidepressant
B   For prevention of bipolar depression a tricyclic antidepressant is better than lithium
C   If a drug fails then electroconvulsive therapy will also fail
D   Most cases of depression recover spontaneously
E   Amphetamine is useful in depression

18.6 Psychotropic drugs may be classified as

A neuroleptics
B anxiolytic sedatives
C antidepressants
D psychostimulants
E psychodysleptics

18.7 In psychiatry

A drug responses are easy to measure
B dosage of drug can be readily and precisely adjusted according to clinical response
C ideal therapeutic response may occur at intermediate plasma concentrations of some antidepressants
D where therapeutic response is difficult to measure it is particularly useful to know the plasma concentration of the drug
E dose increments should be added at intervals that take into account the half-life of the drug

18.8 Actions of neuroleptics include

A dopamine receptor block
B α-adrenoceptor block
C β-adrenoceptor block
D anticholinergic effects
E potentiation of other drugs

18.9 Adverse reactions to phenothiazine neuroleptics include

A cholestatic jaundice
B akathisia
C dry mouth
D parkinsonian syndrome
E tardive dyskinesia

18.10 With injected (i.m.) long-acting depot neuroleptics

A   patient non-compliance is halved
B   defaulters are identifiable
C   hepatic first-pass metabolism is enhanced
D   extrapyramidal syndromes are common and are treated by an anticholinergic drug
E   severe depression can occur

18.11 The following statements about tricyclic antidepressants are correct:

A   Cholinergic side-effects are common
B   Interactions with sympathomimetics and antihypertensives are clinically important
C   To reduce non-compliance it is particularly important to advise depressed patients of even relatively minor adverse effects
D   Overdose carries serious cardiovascular hazard
E   Overdose is readily treated by dialysis because they have a large apparent volume of distribution

18.12 Tricyclic antidepressants

A   can be expected to relieve depression within 48 hours
B   may be given in single evening dose
C   have plasma t½s that vary from 15–200 hours
D   can be effective in nocturnal enuresis in children, but introduce a real risk of poisoning into the home
E   are no use in chronic pain

18.13 When making a choice of antidepressant it is useful to take into account that

A   amitriptyline has sedative effect
B   imipramine has little sedative effect
C   protriptyline has stimulant effect
D   mianserin is comparatively free from cardiotoxic effect
E   mianserin does not antagonise antihypertensives

18.14 **Monoamine oxidase inhibitors of both A and B type**

A   cause decrease in catecholamines and 5-hydroxytryptamine in the central nervous system
B   allow increased absorption of monoamines from the gut
C   allow reduced hepatic first-pass metabolism of monoamines absorbed from the gut
D   potentiate injected sympathomimetics that act directly on adrenoceptors (e.g. adrenaline in local anaesthetic)
E   potentiate injected sympathomimetics that act indirectly by causing release of noradrenaline stores

18.15 **A patient on treatment with a monoamine oxidase inhibitor (A+B) is at risk of a hypertensive reaction if he or she consumes**

A   milk
B   yoghurt
C   butter
D   cheese
E   scrambled egg

18.16 **From knowledge of the mechanism of hypertensive crisis in a patient taking a monoamine oxidase inhibitor it is evident that immediate control of the blood pressure will be achievable with**

A   propranolol
B   methyldopa
C   captopril
D   clonidine
E   phentolamine

18.17 The following statements about lithium are correct:

A Sustained release formulations are particularly to be avoided

B It is distributed throughout body water, ie its apparent volume of distribution is about 50 litres in a 70 kg person

C Its use must be controlled by regular measurement of plasma concentration

D Concomitant use of a diuretic can reduce renal clearance of the drug, causing toxicity

E Its principal use is in prophylaxis of manic-depressive disorder

18.18 Amphetamine

A acts by increasing the amount of noradrenaline stored in nerve endings throughout the nervous system

B excites adults but sedates some hyperactive children

C overdose can cause an acute psychotic state

D overdose can cause hyperthermia

E is useful in narcolepsy

18.19 The following statements about appetite suppressants are correct:

A The use of methylcellulose is preferred above drugs

B They do not induce dependence

C Fenfluramine (Ponderax) is related to amphetamine but acts via serotonin (5HT) rather than noradrenaline

D Fenfluramine antagonises antihypertensive drugs

E They should be used only briefly as their effect is transient

18.20 The following statements about caffeine and caffeine-containing drinks are correct:

A Caffeine is useful primarily to relieve and prevent fatigue

B Caffeine has a t½ of 1 to 2 hours

C Clinically significant overdose of caffeine can occur with amounts in excess of 5 cups of coffee or 10 cups of tea a day

D Caffeine overdose may mimic an anxiety state

E Theophylline has actions similar to caffeine, but its clinical use is as a bronchial relaxant in asthma

19 Central Nervous System IV: Epilepsy: Parkinsonism: Tetanus

19.1 In the management of epilepsy

A all hypnotics and sedatives are useful

B patients must be persuaded of the importance of continuous medication

C treatment must be life long

D it may be possible to discover and eliminate precipitating factors

E the timing of medication should be adjusted if fits occur only at a particular time of day or night

19.2 In the management of epilepsy

A sudden cessation of treatment may result in status epilepticus

B monitoring plasma concentration of drugs is solely a research tool

C the majority of patients can be controlled on a single drug

D the physician needs to know and use the pharmacokinetic properties of each drug prescribed

E most patients can be relieved of their fits within one year of starting treatment

19.3   In epileptic women under treatment

A   there is a threefold increase in the rate of malformations in their children

B   the physiological changes of pregnancy do not alter the pharmacokinetics of antiepilepsy drugs

C   drug therapy should be stopped during pregnancy

D   any malformation in their children is more likely to be due to the disease rather than the drugs

E   some drugs enhance the metabolism of oral contraceptives, when a high dose oestrogen preparation should be used

19.4   In the treatment of epilepsy

A   phenytoin and sodium valproate are first-choice drugs for major seizures

B   ethosuximide is a first-choice drug for minor seizures

C   paraldehyde is the first-choice drug for status epilepticus

D   when the dose is changed some drugs may take a week or more to reach a steady concentration in the plasma

E   adjustments of dosage can reliably be carried out by counting the frequency of fits

19.5   Phenytoin

A   plasma t½ is the same at all plasma concentrations

B   is subject only to first order kinetics

C   enhances its own metabolism

D   is unlikely to cause drug interactions in a patient taking other medication

E   has a remarkably small range of adverse effects

19.6 The following statements about antiepileptic drugs are correct:

A Sodium valproate is a potent hepatic enzyme inducer
B In a patient taking sodium valproate blood coagulation should be examined before surgery is undertaken
C Carbamazepine can be of value in epilepsy even if the patient does not suffer from trigeminal neuralgia as well
D Clonazepam is effective in status epilepticus
E Troxidone is obsolescent because of its adverse reactions

19.7 In Parkinson's disease

A the basal ganglia are deficient in dopamine
B anticholinesterases improve movement
C reserpine replenishes dopamine stores
D chlorpromazine aggravates the condition
E amantadine improves movements by its anticholinergic effect

19.8 Levodopa

A is a metabolic product of dopamine
B penetrates poorly into the central nervous system
C is not metabolised in peripheral tissues
D causes nausea
E causes cardiac dysrhythmias

19.9 The following statements are correct:

A Pyridoxine reduces the therapeutic effect of levodopa used alone but not when it is combined with a decarboxylase inhibitor
B Dangerous hypertension may occur if levodopa is taken with a monamine oxidase Type A inhibitor
C A monoamine oxidase Type B inhibitor (selegiline) usefully prolongs the action of levodopa
D Tricylic antidepressants antagonise the effect of levodopa
E Metabolites of dopamine can interfere with tests for phaeochromocytoma

19.10 Bromocriptine

A is a dopamine antagonist
B has a longer plasma t½ than levodopa
C can cause psychiatric disturbances
D can cause postural hypotension
E is used to initiate lactation

19.11 In the treatment of Parkinson's disease

A anticholinergic drugs are particularly effective in relieving hypokinesia
B levodopa is particularly effective in reducing tremor
C amantadine is as effective as levodopa
D ankle oedema may be caused by amantadine
E haloperidol improves hypokinesia

19.12 In the treatment of Parkinson's disease

A involuntary movements are an indication that too much levodopa is being taken
B postural hypotension due to levodopa may occur
C levodopa initially restores 75% of patients to near normal function
D selegiline helps levodopa 'end-of-dose' akinesia
E the 'on-off' phenomenon is worsened by increasing the frequency of dosing

19.13 The following statements are correct:

A After 10 years of levodopa therapy about 50% of patients experience 'on-off' phenomenon
B Benign essential tremor is alleviated by alcohol
C Intractable hiccup may benefit from chlorpromazine
D Acute dystonic reactions due to neuroleptics should be treated with i.v. levodopa
E Chorea is improved by drugs that reduce the effect of dopamine

19.14 **The following statements about levodopa+dopa decarboxylase inhibitor combinations are correct:**

A It is essential that the decarboxylase inhibitor should enter the central nervous system

B Combinations cause less nausea than does levodopa on its own

C When a decarboxylase inhibitor is added to levodopa, the concentration of levodopa in the brain can be maintained with only one quarter the dose of levodopa used alone

D Decarboxylase inhibitors interfere with active transport of levodopa by the small intestine

E Combinations are safe to use with monoamine oxidase inhibitors

19.15 **In tetanus prophylaxis**

A human tetanus immunoglobulin should be given to all patients with dirty wounds

B a dose of human tetanus immunoglobulin gives reasonable protection for 4 weeks

C injured subjects not known to be actively immune to tetanus should be given a dose of toxoid when seen, as the first dose of a course to be completed later

D toxoid and immunoglobulin (antitoxin) may be mixed in the same syringe

E a booster dose of toxoid is not necessary if the wounded subject has had a full course of toxoid (or a booster dose to a full course) within the past 10 years

19.16 **In clinical tetanus**

A human immunoglobulin is of no value unless given intravenously

B penicillin will not stop further production of toxin

C tetanus spasms may be controlled by diazepam

D chlorpromazine in large doses may make convulsions worse

E treatment with tubocurarine and artificial respiration should be considered where spasms can otherwise only be controlled by making the patient unconscious

20 Central Nervous System V: Non-medical Use of Drugs, Drug Dependence, Tobacco, Alcohol, Cannabis, etc.

20.1 Motives for non-medical drug use include

A relief of anxiety and personal psychological problems
B search for self-knowledge and meaning in life
C conformity with social subgroup
D fun, recreation
E success in sport

20.2 The following statements about non-medical drug use and drug abuse are correct:

A Abuse potential of a drug is related to its capacity to produce immediate satisfaction
B Abuse potential of a drug is uninfluenced by its route of administration
C Drugs that insulate the individual from environmental stress and anxiety are the most likely to be abused
D Drugs that can provide an intense pleasurable experience are particularly likely to be abused
E Multiple drug abuse is common

20.3 **The following statements about non-medical drug use or abuse are correct:**

A Criteria for what constitutes drug abuse are the same for all societies

B It is not the drug alone, but also the way it is used that provides the basis for the classification 'hard' and 'soft'

C Spiritual or religious experience can be regarded as a normal dose-related pharmacodynamic effect of some drugs

D The claim that drugs can provide a basis for a 'culture' may best be judged by results, ie by the contribution of its exponents to society in terms of practice and example

E Even 'soft' use of drugs such as alcohol and tobacco is so potentially hazardous that it should be countered by legislation designed to eliminate them from society

20.4 **The following statements about the use of drugs to gain advantage in sport are correct:**

A Anabolic steroids are used by athletes to improve performance in the 100 metre sprint

B Stimulants such as amphetamine are used to improve performance in weight-lifting

C Detection of drug use is specially difficult where drug or metabolites are closely related to physiological substances

D Caffeine may be taken as diet (coffee) or as medicine (tablets)

E Caffeine can improve physical performance

20.5 **Features of the drug dependent state include**

A emotional distress if the drug is withheld

B physical illness if the drug is withheld

C a need to increase the dose

D continuous use

E intermittent use

20.6 **The following statements about drug dependence and tolerance are correct:**

A Physical dependence is a major factor with cocaine
B Physical dependence is a major factor with opioids
C Cross tolerance between different chemical classes of drug does not occur
D Cross tolerance occurs between members of the same chemical class of drug
E Emotional dependence may occur to any drug that alters consciousness

20.7 **The following statements about drug abuse are correct:**

A Schoolchildren can purchase glues and aerosols without question from the vendor whereas the vendor of alcohol has a motive to refuse sale
B Heroin abuse occurs chiefly amongst teenagers
C Alcohol abuse occurs at any age
D The opinion that 'What a man may lawfully seek in wine surely he may lawfully find in opium' remains as true now as it was in 1821
E Young users of drugs by the intravenous route have a mortality up to 40×normal

20.8 **Established opioid addicts**

A of long standing take the drug *primarily* to avoid the unpleasantness of withdrawal
B who self-inject can easily be transferred to oral methadone since this preparation also provides the sought-after 'kick' or 'high'
C who are in pain from physical injury can be treated satisfactorily by giving a different opioid in ordinary dose
D who self-inject are particularly liable to life-endangering infections and thromboembolism
E who have been subjected to complete drug withdrawal and have regained physical health are not specially prone to relapse

20.9 Morphine-type drug dependence is characterised by

A severe physical dependence
B slight emotional dependence
C marked tolerance
D cross-tolerance with other opioids
E resistance to naloxone

20.10 Barbiturate-type drug dependence is characterised by

A severe emotional dependence
B slight physical dependence
C tolerance
D cross-tolerance with alcohol
E cross-tolerance with benzodiazepines

20.11 The following statements about drug abuse or dependence are correct:

A Cannabis induces marked physical dependence and tolerance
B Tobacco induces severe emotional dependence
C Amphetamine use can cause a psychotic state
D Cocaine induces marked tolerance
E Drug abuse and dependence are primarily pharmacological problems and will be solved by pharmacological research

20.12 The following statements about tobacco smoking are correct:

A Smoke of pipes and cigars is alkaline and therefore nicotine is readily absorbed via the buccal mucosa
B Smoke of cigarettes is acidic and therefore nicotine is not readily absorbed via the buccal mucosa
C Cigarette smokers tend to inhale
D Cigar and pipe smokers tend not to inhale
E Cigarette smokers who inhale may have as much as 15% of their haemoglobin converted to carboxyhaemoglobin

20.13 **The following statements about smoking are correct:**

A Tobacco can be aptly described as 'a pharmacological aid in man's search for contentment'

B Cigarette smokers tend to have introverted rigid personalities

C Sigmund Freud suggested that a powerful motive for smoking might be persistence into adult life of a childhood 'constitutional intensification of the erotogenic significance of the labial region'

D Sigmund Freud did not smoke

E Starting to smoke may be linked with 'self-esteem and status needs'

20.14 **Pharmacological factors involved in smoking include**

A adjustment of plasma nicotine concentration by automatic changes in puffing rate and inhalation

B avoidance of nicotine withdrawal feelings

C a mix of sedative and stimulant action on the central nervous system depending on the psychological state at the time

D increased airways resistance

E no notable cardiovascular effects

20.15 **The following statements about the risks of tobacco smoking are correct:**

A 15% of male non-smokers aged 35 years are dead by age 65 years

B 40% of male smokers of 25 or more cigarettes a day are dead by age 65 years

C Cigarette smoking causes induction of hepatic metabolising enzymes

D The time by which a habitual smoker's life is shortened is about one hour for each cigarette smoked

E The extra death rate of smokers is chiefly the result of cardiovascular and respiratory diseases

20.16 The risk of death from lung cancer is influenced by

A number of cigarettes smoked
B age of starting smoking
C use of filter-tipped cigarettes
D giving up smoking
E use of pipe or cigars

20.17 Smoking is a risk factor for

A coronary heart disease
B increased blood viscosity
C chronic obstructive lung disease
D peptic ulcer
E the unborn child

20.18 The following statements about stopping smoking are correct:

A It is generally easy to stop
B Ex-smoker status is a stable state
C There are no differences between women and men in stopping and staying stopped
D Tranquillisers are important aids in maintaining long-term ex-smoker status
E Nicotine chewing gum allows time-consuming psychosocial approaches, eg group therapy, to be abandoned

20.19 **The following statements about passive smoking are correct:**

A Passive smoking means breathing environmental air contaminated by smoke generated by oneself
B Mainstream and sidestream cigarette smoke have the same composition
C Concentrations of carbon monoxide in the air at a party can be ×4, and in a submarine ×20, those in smoke-free air
D About 10% of non-smokers living in a city have nicotine in their blood
E Children whose parents smoke are more prone to respiratory illness than are those of non-smoking parents

20.20 **Ethyl alcohol (alcohol) characteristically causes**

A loss of finer grades of judgement and attention even at low doses
B loss of power to control mood
C increase in physical efficiency
D peripheral vasoconstriction
E increased secretion of antidiuretic hormone

20.21 **The following statements about alcohol are correct:**

A Gastric acid secretion is first inhibited then increased
B After an initial increase in blood dextrose alcohol causes hypoglycaemia which can be severe
C Vomiting is primarily due to a direct gastric irritant action
D In acute overdose inhalation of vomit is the commonest cause of death
E A pregnant woman who will not abstain should be persuaded to consume less than five units per week

20.22 **Alcohol-dependence is characterised by**

A slight emotional dependence
B trivial physical dependence
C inability to discuss the problem
D absence of tolerance
E surreptitious drinking

20.23 The following statements about alcohol are correct:

  A Alcohol acts in the manner of general inhalation anaesthetics
  B Food, especially milk, delays absorption
  C Habitual drinkers metabolise alcohol more rapidly than non-habitual drinkers
  D It is distributed throughout body water
  E It is subject to saturation or zero-order kinetics

20.24 The following statements about consumption of alcoholic beverages are correct:

  A A woman who consumes more than 2 units daily over a long period (years) exposes herself to liver injury, and with 6 units the risk is grave
  B Per unit dose of alcohol, men develop a higher blood concentration than do women
  C Heavy drinkers develop hepatic cirrhosis at a rate of about 2% per annum
  D There is no biochemical marker for heavy alcohol consumption
  E A standard bottle of spirits (eg gin, whisky) contains more alcohol than an average person can metabolise in 24 hours

20.25 Chronic alcohol dependence is characterised by

  A psychotic states
  B nutritional deficiencies
  C cholestatic hepatitis
  D dementia
  E recovery if the subject stops drinking, even at a late stage

20.26 Acute overdose of alcohol can cause

A excited and violent behaviour which is best controlled by a barbiturate given intramuscularly
B an episode of acute hepatitis
C fall in serum transaminase
D increase in blood clotting factors
E hyperuricaemia and acute gout

20.27 Alcohol (ethanol)

A only affects car driving skills if there is physical inco-ordination of a degree detectable on clinical examination and testing
B causes increased vigilance at low doses
C causes drivers to have accidents with other cars on the road but to be able to drive safely when there is no other traffic
D induces overconfidence
E reduces reaction time

20.28 Methyl alcohol (methanol)

A is sometimes drunk as a substitute for ethyl alcohol
B has a time-course of intoxication similar to that of ethyl alcohol
C causes intense acidosis
D overdose is treated by sodium bicarbonate and ethyl alcohol
E poisoning may cause permanent blindness

20.29 The following statement about psychodysleptics and hallucinogens (lysergide or LSD, mescaline etc.) are correct:

A   They have no proved therapeutic use

B   Their actions cannot be described as precisely as is possible for most other drugs since their effects are highly conditioned by the subject's frame of mind, personality and environment

C   They do not cause psychotic reactions

D   Physical dependence occurs

E   'Bad trips' may be treated with diazepam or chlorpromazine

20.30 When cannabis is taken

A   tolerance does not occur

B   memory and attention are impaired and the subject becomes more suggestible

C   cannabinoids are taken up in body fat and slowly released

D   vasodilation and tachycardia are usual

E   psychotic reactions do not occur

21 Anaesthesia and Neuromuscular Block

21.1 The following statements about stages of anaesthesia are correct:

A In Stage 1 sense of touch is retained and sense of hearing increased

B In Stage 2 delirium precedes unconsciousness

C In surgical anaesthesia (Stage 3) the corneal reflex does not disappear until plane IV

D Some degree of medullary paralysis occurs at all planes of Stage 3

E Stages 1 and 2 are hardly recognisable with modern techniques

21.2 The responsibility of the anaesthetist

A begins immediately before surgery when the patient arrives at the operating theatre

B is concerned with the patient's physical but not psychological condition

C requires that he be informed of all drugs the patient may be receiving

D involves providing unconsciousness, analgesia and muscular relaxation with a single drug whenever this is possible

E ceases when patient leaves the operating theatre

21.3 Anaesthetic premedication involves considerations of providing

A alertness
B amnesia
C analgesia
D stimulation of the autonomic nervous system
E a satisfactory postsurgical state

21.4 A typical anaesthetic for abdominal surgery includes

A gradual induction by an inhaled agent
B maintenance by an agent given intravenously
C analgesia by increasing the concentration of the inhaled agent
D muscular relaxation with tubocurarine
E the provision of apparatus for mechanically assisted respiration

21.5 After an abdominal operation the anaesthetist

A may need to use antagonists to neuromuscular blocking agents
B must not leave patients alone until they are conscious
C plays a role in relief of postoperative pain
D should ensure that the cough reflex is fully suppressed
E cannot be expected to prevent postoperative vomiting

21.6 The single-handed operator-anaesthetist

A should make sure the patient is unconscious
B may employ 'dissociative' anaesthesia
C may employ 'neuroleptanalgesia'
D may employ paraldehyde for procedures where there is no pain eg endoscopy
E obliged to use an inhalation agent should prefer ether to halothane

21.7   **The following statements about the kinetics of inhalation anaesthetics are correct:**

A   An agent that is highly soluble in blood, given at constant rate, provides a slow induction
B   An agent that is relatively insoluble in blood, given at constant rate, provides a fast induction
C   Nitrous oxide provides slow induction
D   Diffusion anoxia occurs particularly with nitrous oxide when the agent is withdrawn
E   Recovery from anaesthesia is fast if the agent is relatively insoluble in blood

21.8   **Intravenous anaesthetics**

A   provide slow induction
B   provide particularly quick recovery even after prolonged use
C   depend for their duration of effect on redistribution of drug in the body
D   depending on metabolism for their elimination can be expected to have a short duration of action
E   can cause loss of the arm if injected by mistake into the brachial artery

21.9   **The following statements about ether and nitrous oxide are correct:**

A   In ether overdose cessation of respiration occurs before cardiac arrest
B   The use of ether is declining because it is flammable and induction is slow
C   After even prolonged ether anaesthesia the postoperative recovery period is not unpleasant
D   Nitrous oxide cannot alone maintain surgical anaesthesia
E   In obstetrics a self-administered mixture of nitrous oxide 80%, oxygen 20% provides efficient and safe analgesia

21.10 Halothane

A provides quick induction and recovery
B causes hypotension and cardiac dysrhythmias
C may cause jaundice if given repeatedly in the course of a few weeks.
D should not be used if previous use has been followed by unexplained fever
E does not induce hepatic drug metabolising enzymes

21.11 Thiopentone

A provides singularly unpleasant induction
B causes sudden apnoea if injected rapidly
C does not often cause laryngospasm
D has a plasma t½ of 2.5 minutes in the early phase of an injection
E has a plasma t½ of 2 hours after equilibration

21.12 Neuromuscular blocking drug action is

A by competition
B by depolarisation
C by blocking autonomic ganglia
D reversible by an anticholinesterase in the case of suxamethonium
E reversible by chlorpromazine in the case of tubocurarine

21.13 Neuromuscular blocking drugs

A are used to provide muscular relaxation with only light anaesthesia by central nervous system depressants
B carry no risk of awareness during surgery
C are sufficiently selective to allow spontaneous respiration to be maintained in many cases
D acting by competition are preferred for long procedures
E acting by depolarisation do not cause postoperative muscle pain

21.14 Neuromuscular blocking agents are useful in therapy of

 A myasthenia gravis
 B status epilepticus
 C spastic paraplegia
 D tetanus
 E electroconvulsive therapy (ECT)

21.15 Centrally-acting muscle relaxants, eg baclofen

 A do not cause objectionable sedation
 B improve voluntary motor power
 C may make the patient worse even if spasticity in the legs is reduced
 D control flexor spasms
 E require provision of artificial respiration

21.16 A desirable local anaesthetic should

 A be non-irritant to tissues
 B have a slow onset of action
 C be soluble in water
 D be sterilisable by heat
 E have a built-in vasodilator action

21.17 Local anaesthetics

 A act by altering ionic permeability of nerve cell membranes
 B prevent initiation and propagation of the nerve impulse
 C may be absorbed sufficiently to cause systemic toxicity
 D affect first the larger (motor) nerve fibres and last the small (sensory) fibres
 E are all absorbed across mucous membranes

21.18 Local anaesthetic

A action may be prolonged by addition of a vasodilator
B application to extremities (eg toe) should always be conducted with added adrenaline
C mixed with adrenaline may cause severe hypertension in a patient taking a monoamine oxidase inhibitor
D mixed with adrenaline may cause severe hypertension in a patient taking a tricyclic antidepressant
E mixed with felypressin is preferable in patients with cardiovascular disease

21.19 Local anaesthetics

A are usually effective within one minute of application
B have a useful duration of action of 1–2 hours
C are most stable in the form of acid salts
D have an enhanced action in inflamed tissues
E are absorbed and metabolised in the liver

21.20 Local anaesthetic

A overdose can cause convulsions
B overdose can cause cardiovascular collapse
C may be applied to a surface
D may be infiltrated around the lesion
E must never be infiltrated around major peripheral nerves or near the spinal cord

21.21 Lignocaine

A is useful in cardiac dysrhythmias
B is less toxic than prilocaine in overdose
C unlike prilocaine, is not effective when applied to mucous membranes
D differs structurally from most other local anaesthetics
E carries no risk of convulsions in overdose

21.22 Cocaine

A   is effective on mucous membranes
B   enhances natural catecholamine effects
C   is not absorbed across mucous membranes
D   is abused for its central nervous system stimulation
E   overdose should be treated by adrenoceptor blocking drugs

21.23 The following statements about the use of drugs in childbirth are correct:

A   Pethidine depresses fetal respiration more than morphine
B   Naloxone antagonises both morphine and pethidine
C   Nitrous oxide is a potent fetal respiratory depressant despite its brief action
D   Diazepam dose must be carefully restricted as it is capable of depressing the newborn baby for several days
E   Vasoconstrictors can cause fetal distress by reducing placental blood flow

21.24 When drugs are used in childbirth

A   it is important to work out a schedule of drug dosage in advance and not to be diverted from it
B   opioids delay gastric emptying
C   a dose of metoclopramide will ensure an empty stomach in a patient who has received pethidine, if emergency general anaesthesia is needed
D   neuromuscular blocking agents must be avoided in Caesarian section
E   gastric antacids and histamine H_2-receptor blocking drugs have no role

21.25 **The following statements about the interaction of anaesthetics with other drugs are correct:**

A   A patient taking a monoamine oxidase inhibitor may be premedicated with morphine

B   A patient under treatment for hypertension is liable to hypotension during general anaesthesia

C   Oral contraceptives predispose to postoperative thromboembolism

D   Diuretic-induced hypokalaemia potentiates neuromuscular blocking drugs

E   Aminoglycoside antibiotics antagonise neuromuscular blocking drugs

21.26 **Special care before and during general anaesthesia is required in patients having**

A   fixed cardiac output

B   renal failure

C   myasthenia gravis

D   porphyria

E   diabetes mellitus

21.27 **Factors which may influence the normal response to anaesthesia include**

A   hypothyroidism

B   malignant hyperthermia

C   sickle-cell disease

D   the age of the patient

E   atmospheric pollution of the operating theatre

22 Cholinergic and Anticholinergic Drugs

22.1 **The following statements about cholinergic agents are correct:**

A The actions of acetylcholine at autonomic ganglia and the neuromuscular junction are described as nicotinic
B Pilocarpine inhibits cholinesterase
C Physostigmine acts selectively at end-organs that respond to acetylcholine
D Carbachol has more prominent muscarinic than nicotinic effects
E Cholinergic drugs cause bronchodilation

22.2 **The following statements about cholinergic agents are correct:**

A Pilocarpine has a clinically useful miotic action
B Pilocarpine may be used to stimulate salivary flow in patients taking large doses of an anticholinergic drug
C Carbachol is safe to give intravenously
D Cholinergic drugs cause muscle fasciculation
E *Amanita muscaria* was highly valued by ancient Vikings for its cerebral stimulant effects

22.3 **Cholinergic stimulation causes**

A intraocular pressure to rise
B sweating
C tachycardia
D reduced gut motility
E contraction of the bladder

22.4 **The following statements about anticholinesterases are correct:**

A Pseudocholinesterases metabolise substances other than acetylcholine

B Physostigmine lowers intra-ocular pressure

C Neostigmine may be used with atropine to reverse competitive neuromuscular block

D Pyridostigmine may have fewer visceral effects than neostigmine

E Edrophonium has a long duration of action

22.5 **In anticholinesterase poisoning**

A due to organophosphorus insecticides, inhibition of cholinesterase is irreversible and recovery depends on formation of fresh enzyme

B bronchoconstriction may occur

C atropine should be used sparingly

D due to organophosphorus insecticides, treatment with pralidoxime should be delayed for 24 h

E recovery of plasma cholinesterase may take several weeks

22.6 **In myasthenia gravis**

A neostigmine given for diagnostic purposes should be accompanied by atropine to suppress unwanted visceral (muscarinic) effects

B if the daily dose of anticholinesterase is less than 15 tablets and the pupil diameter exceeds 3 mm, weakness is likely to be due to excess of cholinergic action

C weakness that increases more than 2 h after a dose and is relieved by the next dose is probably myasthenic

D edrophonium exaggerates a myasthenic crisis and alleviates a cholinergic crisis

E habitual use of atropine may mask excessive therapy

22.7 In myasthenia gravis

A forcing the dose of anticholinesterase drug to correct diplopia may cause a cholinergic crisis

B pyridostigmine is usually preferred as its action is smoother than that of neostigmine

C thymectomy is effective in patients under 40 years who do not have a thymoma

D prednisolone induces improvement or remission in 80% of cases

E prednisolone is contraindicated when the disease is predominantly ocular

22.8 Atropine

A antagonises all the effects of cholinergic drugs except those at autonomic ganglia and the neuromuscular junction

B promotes sweating

C relaxes smooth muscle

D is used to treat glaucoma

E inhibits milk production

22.9 Atropine

A administered to the eye may interfere with normal pupillary responses for up to 2 weeks

B reduces the heart rate

C loosens viscid bronchial secretions

D may induce urinary retention

E prevents and suppresses motion sickness

22.10 Features of atropine poisoning include

A mydriasis

B hallucinations

C hypothermia

D coma

E dry mouth

22.11 Anticholinergic drugs may be used to treat

A asthma
B colic
C urinary urgency incontinence
D vomiting
E heart block

23 Cardiovascular System I: Adrenergic Mechanisms: Sympathomimetic Agents

23.1 The following statements about the effects of adrenaline and noradrenaline are correct:

A The classification of adrenoceptors is based on the observation that block of the whole range of actions of adrenaline could not be attained by a single drug

B There are two major classes of adrenoceptor

C α-adrenoceptor blocking drugs block the cardiac and vasodilator effects of adrenaline

D β-adrenoceptor blocking drugs block the vasoconstrictor effect of adrenaline and noradrenaline

E Relaxation of the smooth muscle of the bronchi and uterus is mediated by β-adrenoceptors

23.2 Drugs may mimic or impair adrenergic mechanisms by

A binding directly onto adrenoceptors

B discharging noradrenaline stored in nerve endings

C preventing reuptake into nerve endings of noradrenaline that has been released

D preventing destruction of noradrenaline in the nerve ending

E depleting noradrenaline stores in nerve endings

23.3 Drugs may mimic or impair adrenergic mechanisms by

A causing the nerve ending to synthesise a false transmitter

B acting in the central nervous system

C acting at parasympathetic nerve terminals

D acting as first messengers at adrenoceptors

E acting as second messengers at adrenoceptors

23.4 Physiological events mediated by α-adrenoceptors include

A increased heart rate
B hypokalaemia
C peripheral arteriolar constriction
D bronchoconstriction
E cardiac dysrhythmia

23.5 Physiological events mediated by β-adrenoceptors include

A mydriasis
B peripheral arteriolar dilation
C relaxation of pregnant myometrium
D voluntary muscle tremor
E increased myocardial contractility

23.6 The following statements about the action of sympathomimetics are correct:

A Adrenaline has almost exclusively β-adrenoceptor agonist actions
B Noradrenaline has an approximately equal mix of α-and β-adrenoceptor agonist actions
C Isoprenaline has predominantly α-adrenoceptor agonist actions
D Amphetamine acts indirectly by causing release of noradrenaline stored in nerve endings
E Dopamine acts not only on specific dopamine receptors but also on adrenoceptors

23.7 Catecholamines comprise

A adrenaline
B noradrenaline
C dopamine
D dobutamine
E salbutamol

23.8 Catecholamines

A are destroyed by monoamine oxidase
B released at nerve endings are at once destroyed by catechol-O-methyltransferase
C are normally administered by mouth
D have a t½ of one to two minutes
E may be administered i.m. or i.v.

23.9 The following statements about the action of sympathomimetics (i.v.) are correct:

A Noradrenaline infusion causes a rise of systolic and diastolic blood pressure with bradycardia
B Adrenaline infusion causes a rise of systolic and fall of diastolic blood pressure with tachycardia
C Isoprenaline or isoxsuprine cause little change in systolic and fall in diastolic blood pressure with tachycardia and uterine relaxation
D Dopamine causes cardiac stimulation with overall slight reduction in total peripheral resistance and increased renal blood flow
E Dobutamine has greater inotropic than chronotropic effects on the heart

23.10 Shock

A is a state of peripheral vascular hypoperfusion causing anoxic injury to vital organs
B may be caused by infections
C may be caused by loss of fluid from the circulation
D may be caused by cardiac damage
E is treated primarily by getting the blood pressure into the normal range by increasing peripheral vascular resistance with vasoconstrictor drugs

23.11 **In a case of shock, when the patient's needs have been carefully defined, the following statements are correct:**

A   It may be useful to reduce peripheral vascular resistance by an α-adrenoceptor blocking drug

B   Gelatin and hetastarch may be used to restore lost intravascular volume

C   Dopamine provides a mix of adrenergic actions on heart and circulation that is least likely to do harm and may even do good

D   Atropine relieves harmful bradycardia

E   Enormous doses of adrenocortical steroid are life-saving in septic shock

24 Cardiovascular System II: Drugs Used in Arterial Hypertension and Angina Pectoris

24.1 Clinically useful arterial antihypertensive drugs may produce their effects by actions on

A arteriole resistance vessels
B venule capacitance vessels
C adrenal cortex
D central nervous system
E blood volume

24.2 Arterial antihypertensive drugs act on

A parasympathetic ganglia
B α-adrenoceptors
C β-adrenoceptors
D noradrenaline synthesis
E noradrenaline release

24.3 Angiotensin converting enzyme (ACE) inhibitors, eg captopril, enalapril

A block the alteration of inactive angiotensin I to active angiotensin II
B oppose the vasoconstrictor effect of angiotensin II
C stimulate renal aldosterone production
D are useless in heart failure
E are useful in hypertension

24.4   The following statements about arterial antihypertensive and vasodilator drugs are correct:

A   The objective of using antihypertensives is to interfere with homeostatic mechanisms that regulate the blood pressure
B   Antihypertensives that allow drop of pressure in response to erect posture and exercise are preferred
C   Diuretics reduce blood volume but also reduce peripheral arteriolar resistance
D   Dilatation of capacitance vessels reduces cardiac output
E   Reduction of sympathetic autonomic drive to the heart raises cardiac output

24.5   Glyceryl trinitrate

A   relieves an attack of angina pectoris by dilating the venous and arteriolar systems
B   may be substituted by isosorbide mononitrate for prophylaxis of angina pectoris
C   action lasts about 4 hours
D   should be given at once if myocardial infarction is suspected
E   induces tolerance

24.6   When glyceryl trinitrate tablets are prescribed for angina pectoris the patient should be told

A   to take it to prevent pain
B   to take it at onset of pain
C   that if throbbing headache and palpitations occur the patient should take another
D   that if he feels faint he should stand perfectly still and as relaxed as he can
E   to keep the tablets in a warm humid place eg a shelf over the bath

24.7 Glyceryl trinitrate may usefully be taken as

A a sublingual tablet
B a tablet to swallow
C an oral mucosal spray
D an ointment
E a suppository

24.8 The following vasodilator drugs are useful in angina pectoris:

A Angiotensin converting enzyme inhibitor (eg captopril)
B Calcium channel blocker (eg nifedipine)
C Diazoxide
D Hydralazine
E Propranolol

24.9 Diazoxide

A is a thiazide
B is a diuretic
C is a vasodilator
D is extensively bound to plasma protein
E should be given intravenously very slowly because it binds to plasma protein so readily

24.10 Diazoxide

A is useful for long term control of hypertension
B causes sodium retention
C is particularly useful for hypertension during childbirth (labour)
D is useful in hypoglycaemia due to pancreatic β-islet cell tumours
E acts on arterioles (cardiac afterload) rather than on veins (cardiac preload)

24.11 Hydralazine

A dilates veins rather than arterioles
B does not generally cause postural hypotension
C is particularly suitable for sole treatment of hypertension
D characteristically causes bradycardia
E is acetylated in the body and patients may be classed as slow and fast metabolisers

24.12 In heart failure (acute or chronic) vasodilators

A can usefully be added to a diuretic
B relieve cardiac preload
C relieve cardiac afterload
D usefully reduce cardiac output
E that are used include organic nitrates and sodium nitroprusside

24.13 In obstructive peripheral vascular disease

A drug therapy is more likely to be beneficial in arteriosclerosis than in vascular spasm
B if the skin of the leg becomes warmer it can be assumed flow to the muscles is similarly improved
C nocturnal muscle cramps occur and may be relieved by quinine
D a β-adrenoceptor blocker benefits
E any benefit may be due to metabolic changes in the muscle rather than to vasodilatation

24.14 The following statements about α-adrenoceptor blocking drugs are correct:

A They act by competition
B They cause peripheral vasodilatation
C Those that block α_1 and α_2-adrenoceptors are associated with troublesome tachycardia
D Prazosin is preferred in the treatment of hypertension because it selectively blocks α_1-receptors
E Labetalol has both α- and β-adrenoceptor blocking actions

24.15 β-adrenoceptor blocking drugs cause

A reduction of heart rate
B increased myocardial contractility
C reduced peripheral blood flow
D bronchoconstriction
E reduced hepatic blood flow

24.16 β-adrenoceptor blocking drugs

A increase myocardial oxygen consumption
B may have agonist effect in addition to their antagonist effect
C may have a quinidine-like effect
D characteristically lower the blood pressure immediately on commencing therapy
E selective for cardiac β_1-receptors can safely be used in asthmatics

24.17 β-adrenoceptor blocking drugs that are lipid soluble

A have a longer t½ than those that are water soluble
B are extensively subject to hepatic first pass metabolism
C show less predictable plasma concentrations than do those that are water soluble
D are preferred if there is renal insufficiency
E less commonly cause nightmares than do those that are water soluble

24.18 β-adrenoceptor blocking drugs are used in

A arterial hypertension
B anxiety
C hypothyroidism
D cardiac dysrhythmias
E glaucoma

24.19 Patients taking a β-adrenoceptor blocking drug may experience

A exacerbation of existing heart block
B precipitation of heart failure where cardiac performance is dependent on sympathetic drive
C incapacity for vigorous exercise
D cold extremities
E hypoglycaemia if they are diabetic

24.20 The following statements about adrenergic neurone blocking drugs are correct:

A They diminish noradrenaline release from sympathetic nerve endings
B They diminish noradrenaline reuptake into sympathetic nerves
C Tricyclic antidepressants reverse their antihypertensive effect
D Fenfluramine reverses their hypotensive effect
E A characteristic adverse effect is failure of male ejaculation

24.21 The following statements about antihypertensives are correct:

A Reserpine increases noradrenaline stores in nerve endings
B Reserpine is used in combination with a diuretic in hypertension
C Metyrosine prevents conversion of tyrosine to dopa and has a place in treatment of phaeochromocytoma
D Trimetaphan is not used for producing controlled hypotension in surgery because it causes constipation
E Ganglion-blocking drugs are insufficiently selective for long-term use as antihypertensives

24.22 Clonidine

  A acts on β-adrenoceptors in the brain
  B acts on presynaptic α₂-adrenoceptors at the sympathetic nerve ending
  C causes marked postural hypotension
  D withdrawal, if sudden, may be followed by dangerous hypertension
  E has a reputation for prophylactic efficacy in menopausal flushing and migraine

24.23 Methyldopa

  A probably acts by causing the formation of a false sympathetic transmitter
  B is relatively free from unwanted postural hypotension
  C causes hyperactive behaviour
  D causes a positive Coomb's test with, occasionally, haemolytic anaemia
  E causes depression

24.24 Angina pectoris may benefit from:

  A drugs which interfere with passage of calcium into cells: calcium antagonists
  B vasodilators
  C stopping smoking
  D α-adrenoceptor block
  E β-adrenoceptor block

24.25 **The following statements about treatment of arterial hypertension are correct:**

A Blood pressure measurement is objective and drug trials do not require placebo use or double blind technique

B The objective of treatment is to stabilise the blood pressure at about 165/95 mm Hg

C Elderly people especially require urgent reduction of blood pressure

D Treatment should be given even in the absence of symptoms

E Women are particularly vulnerable to the consequences of hypertension

24.26 **In the control of arterial hypertension**

A where a single drug is used there is a tendency for homeostatic adjustments to annul its effect

B drug combinations, where each drug acts at a different site, improve efficacy

C drug combinations, where each drug acts at a different site, reduce the incidence of unwanted effects

D even mild cases require a drug combination from the start

E guanethidine and methyldopa are drugs of choice for mild cases

24.27 **Long term diuretic use can cause**

A hyperkalaemia

B impaired male sexual function

C impaired glucose tolerance

D gout

E Raynaud's phenomenon

24.28 **In the emergency control of severe arterial hypertension by parenteral therapy**

A propranolol is best
B labetalol is effective
C hydralazine is effective
D sodium nitroprusside is effective
E reduction of pressure by more than 25% over minutes may cause cerebral infarction

24.29 **The following statements are correct:**

A In hypertension of pregnancy, a diuretic is preferred
B In hypertension of pregnancy, methyldopa is acceptable
C In hypertension of pregnancy, a β-adrenoceptor blocker is acceptable
D Non-steroidal anti-inflammatory drugs potentiate the effect of diuretics and β-adrenoceptor blockers
E Prophylactic glyceryl trinitrate may be useful to avoid an attack of angina pectoris during sexual intercourse

24.30 **The following statements about phaeochromocytoma are correct:**

A Hypertension is sustained, never intermittent
B In a hypertensive emergency a β-adrenoceptor blocking drug must be given first
C In a hypertensive emergency phentolamine is a drug of choice
D Preoperative treatment with both α- and β-adrenoceptor blockade should be given for several days
E An α-adrenoceptor blocking drug can be helpful in diagnosis

25 Cardiovascular System III: Cardiac Dysrhythmia and Cardiac Failure

25.1 The following statements about cardiac cells are correct:

A The atrioventricular node discharges automatically 45 times per minute

B Myocardial muscle cells discharge automatically 25 times per minute

C Altered rate of automatic discharge may be a cause of cardiac dysrhythmia

D In its *phases of polarisation*, the cardiac cell is hyperexcitable during phases 1 and 2

E Cardiac dysrhythmia may result from impaired conduction leading to the formation of re-entry circuits

25.2 The following statements about the classification of antidysrhythmic drugs are correct:

A Class 1 drugs possess membrane stabilising activity

B Class 1A drugs shorten refractoriness

C Class 1B drugs lengthen refractoriness

D Class II drugs block slow calcium channels

E Class III drugs reduce the activity of the sympathetic nervous system

25.3 Quinidine

A prolongs the cardiac refractory period

B prolongs the QT interval of the ECG

C is used to prevent ventricular tachycardia

D lowers plasma digoxin concentration

E causes diarrhoea

25.4 Procainamide

A possesses membrane stabilising activity
B prolongs the cardiac refractory period
C is contraindicated after a myocardial infarction
D is more likely to cause a systemic lupus-like syndrome in slow acetylators
E can cause hypotension

25.5 Disopyramide

A possesses membrane stabilising activity
B prolongs the cardiac refractory period
C is contraindicated for patients with Wolff-Parkinson-White syndrome
D has a positive inotropic effect
E should be avoided in patients with glaucoma

25.6 Lignocaine

A possesses membrane stabilising activity
B reduces the cardiac refractory period
C is not given orally because it is not absorbed from the gastrointestinal tract
D is particularly effective for supraventricular dysrhythmias
E in standard doses achieves higher blood concentrations in patients with cardiac failure than in patients without cardiac failure

25.7 The following statements about cardiac antidysrhythmic drugs are correct:

A Mexiletine has a membrane stabilising activity
B Mexiletine is used for ventricular dysrhythmias
C Phenytoin is contraindicated in cardiac dysrhythmias associated with digoxin overdose
D Flecainide is used mainly for ventricular dysrhythmias
E Sotalol has membrane stabilising activity

25.8 **The following statements about cardiac antidysrhythmic drugs are correct:**

A Practolol should not be used for the emergency treatment of cardiac dysrhythmias because it causes the oculomucocutaneous syndrome

B Propranolol in overdose causes heart block

C Amiodarone has an unusually short plasma t½

D Thyroid function should be checked before a patient begins treatment with amiodarone

E Effects of warfarin are increased in patients who receive amiodarone

25.9 **The following statements about calcium channel blocking drugs are correct:**

A Verapamil has a positive inotropic effect

B Verapamil dilates coronary arteries that are in spasm

C Verapamil effectively relieves atrioventricular block

D Diltiazem may cause ankle oedema

E Nifedipine is contraindicated in Raynaud's disease

25.10 **Stimulation of the vagus nerve**

A causes tachycardia due to its effect on the sino-atrial node

B accelerates conduction in the atrioventricular tissue

C reduces cardiac contractility

D shortens the refractory period of atrial muscle

E decreases myocardial excitability

25.11 **Reflex stimulation of the vagus nerve that is both safe and clinically useful may be produced by**

A eyeball pressure

B pressing on both carotid sinuses simultaneously

C Valsalva's manoeuvre

D the Muller procedure

E inviting the patient to put his fingers down his throat

25.12 Stimulation of the sympathetic nervous system causes

A tachycardia due to increased rate of discharge of the sinoatrial node
B increased conductivity in the His-Purkinje system
C decrease in force of cardiac contraction
D shortening in the cardiac refractory period
E reduced automaticity of the heart

25.13 Digitalis glycosides in therapeutic doses

A increase the excitability of the myocardium
B increase the contractility of the myocardium
C increase generation and propagation of impulses in the sinoatrial and atrioventricular nodes and conducting tissue
D shorten the PR interval on the ECG
E increase T wave amplitude on the ECG

25.14 Digoxin

A has its action terminated mainly by metabolism in the liver
B has a plasma t½ of 6 h
C provides benefit in atrial fibrillation by increasing the force of cardiac contraction
D is of special value in heart failure due to chronic cor pulmonale
E should be given in lower than normal doses to hypothyroid patients

25.15 When administering digoxin

A the loading dose should be the same whether it is given intravenously or orally
B about one third of the loading dose, given daily, should suffice as the maintenance dose
C steady state plasma concentration should be attained within 3 days if a constant daily dose is given
D note should be taken of a complaint of anorexia which may be a warning that the dose is too high
E a steady state plasma concentration of 0.5µg/l is an indication that the dose is too high

25.16 Digoxin toxicity

A is strongly suggested by an ectopic dysrhythmia accompanied by heart block
B is more likely in the elderly
C cannot be held responsible for diarrhoea
D may explain gynaecomastia
E may explain mental confusion

25.17 Digoxin

A should be given in a lower dose if verapamil is also administered
B overdose responds well to treatment by dialysis
C overdose causing dysrhythmia responds well to direct current shock
D overdose may be treated by infusion of specific digoxin-binding antibody fragments
E toxicity causing increased ventricular excitability should be treated with potassium, even in the absence of hypokalaemia

25.18 The principal site of antidysrhythmic action of

A β-adrenoceptor blockers is on the ventricle
B digoxin is on the sinoatrial node, the atrium and the atrioventricular node
C verapamil is on the sinoatrial node, the atrium and the atrioventricular node
D atropine is on the ventricle
E mexiletine is on the atrium

25.19 Paroxysmal atrial and nodal tachycardia

A may be terminated by vagal stimulation
B if accompanied by atrioventricular block should be treated with verapamil
C if recurrent may be prevented with digoxin
D may be due to thyrotoxicosis
E if recurrent may be prevented with a β-adrenoceptor blocker

25.20 Atrial flutter or fibrillation

A in general should be converted to sinus rhythm using direct current shock rather than drugs

B due to long-standing rheumatic mitral valve disease is suitable for attempted conversion to sinus rhythm

C if treated with quinidine alone may give rise to a dangerous increase in ventricular rate

D is corrected safely by direct current shock even if the dysrhythmia is due to digoxin overdose

E with rapid ventricular response should be controlled with digoxin if sinus rhythm cannot be restored

25.21 The following statements about cardiac dysrhythmia are correct:

A Atrial ectopic beats may respond to reduction in intake of xanthine-containing drinks

B In heart block atropine can provide temporary relief

C Digoxin is the drug of choice for supraventricular tachycardia associated with the Wolff-Parkinson-White syndrome

D Lignocaine is effective in suppressing ventricular premature beats after myocardial infarction

E Amiodarone is effective treatment for recurrent ventricular tachycardia

25.22 In cardiac arrest

A the organ most sensitive to anoxia is the heart

B electrocardiographic evidence of asystole is mandatory before starting treatment

C the neck should be fully flexed to aid respiration

D the femoral and carotid pulses should be checked to assess the adequacy of external cardiac massage

E if asystole is present inject calcium chloride intravenously

25.23 In cardiac failure

A dilation of the heart helps temporarily to sustain cardiac output

B the heart and brain receive blood diverted from the liver, kidneys and skin

C activation of the renin-angiotensin-aldosterone system causes peripheral vasoconstriction

D diuretics lower excessive venous filling pressure

E nitrates stimulate myocardial contraction

25.24 In cardiac failure

A hydralazine reduces peripheral vascular resistance

B captopril should be started immediately in full dose

C prazosin dilates arterioles and veins

D dopamine has a positive inotropic effect

E dopamine causes renal cortical vasoconstriction

26 Cardiovascular System IV: Hyperlipidaemias

26.1 In hyperlipidaemia

A Types I, III and V are commoner than Types II and IV

B the biochemical diagnosis should be made on a blood sample taken after a 14 h fast

C clofibrate helps to prevent the formation of gallstones

D clofibrate inhibits hepatic lipid synthesis

E a high alcohol intake is probably associated with the development of some Types

26.2 In the treatment of hyperlipidaemia

A diet alone cannot be expected to produce improvement

B the presence of diabetes mellitus should not be allowed to delay the start of treatment by clofibrate

C cholestyramine may interfere with the absorption of warfarin

D cholestyramine binds bile acids in the intestine

E nicotinic acid derivatives reduce the supply of free fatty acid substrates for hepatic lipoprotein synthesis

27 Kidney and Urinary Tract

27.1 The following statements about renal physiology are correct:

A Each day the body produces a maximum of 20 l of glomerular filtrate

B 65% of filtered sodium is reabsorbed isotonically by the proximal tubule

C Chloride is actively transported from the tubular fluid to the interstitial fluid in the thick segment of the ascending limb of the Loop of Henle

D Interstitial fluid tonicity is high in the cortex and low in the medulla

E The descending limb of the Loop of Henle is impermeable to water

27.2 Diuresis may result from

A increase in cardiac output

B intravenous infusion of a low molecular weight non-electrolyte hypertonic solution

C inhibition of antidiuretic hormone secretion

D drug action on renal glomeruli

E stimulation of renal tubular carbonic anhydrase

27.3   In the kidney diuretic drugs act at the

A   proximal tubule by inhibiting active reabsorption of chloride

B   ascending limb of the Loop of Henle by inhibiting active transport of water

C   cortical diluting segment by preventing sodium reabsorption

D   distal tubule by inhibiting the action of antidiuretic hormone

E   collecting tubule by inhibiting the action of aldosterone

27.4   The principal renal site of action of

A   triamterene is in the ascending limb of the Loop of Henle

B   spironolactone is in the descending limb of the Loop of Henle

C   frusemide is in the proximal tubule

D   osmotic diuretics is in the distal tubule

E   thiazides is in the cortical diluting segment

27.5   The following statements about the action of diuretics in the kidney are correct:

A   Loop diuretics diminish the osmotic gradient between medulla and cortex

B   Diuretics that act in the Loop of Henle have a lower maximal effect than do drugs that act on the cortical diluting segment

C   Diuretics that act in the cortical diluting segment increase the osmotic gradient between medulla and cortex

D   Diuretics that act in the distal tubule have a weak natriuretic effect

E   Thiazides usually remain effective even at glomerular filtration rates below 20 ml/min

27.6   Diuretic drugs may be used to treat

    A   angioedema
    B   hypercalcaemia
    C   idiopathic hypercalciuria
    D   the syndrome of inappropriate antidiuretic hormone secretion
    E   nephrogenic diabetes insipidus

27.7   The following statements about the high efficacy diuretics are correct:

    A   Frusemide is effective when the glomerular filtration rate is less than 10ml/min
    B   Part of the effect of frusemide in relieving acute pulmonary oedema is due to vasodilatation
    C   The diuretic action of a single dose of bumetanide lasts 24 hours
    D   Bumetanide may cause muscle pains in high dosage
    E   Piretanide relaxes vascular smooth muscle

27.8   Thiazide diuretics

    A   are preferred to the loop diuretics for the treatment of hypertension
    B   that are lipid soluble act for longer than those that are water soluble
    C   are uricosuric
    D   may cause thrombocytopenia
    E   are effective antihypertensives partly due to reduction of peripheral vascular resistance

27.9 **The following statements about potassium-sparing diuretics are correct:**

A Spironolactone has low therapeutic efficacy
B Spironolactone may cause gynaecomastia
C Spironolactone may cause hyperkalaemia in patients whose renal function is impaired
D Spironolactone may usefully be combined with triamterene
E Amiloride antagonises the action of aldosterone

27.10 **Potassium depletion**

A with loop diuretics is less than with thiazides for equivalent natriuretic effect
B is revealed by increasing amplitude of the T wave of the ECG
C may be a complication of liquorice used as a confection
D with thiazides is so common that all hypertensives treated with these drugs should receive potassium supplements
E may occur with diarrhoea

27.11 **Potassium replacement**

A with potassium chloride is preferred, especially when high efficacy diuretics are used
B using tablets may result in oesophageal ulceration
C is better retained if it is not given at the same time as the diuretic that is causing the loss
D is essential if amiloride is used
E where a diuretic is used to treat hypertension may be unnecessary if dietary intake of potassium is good

27.12 **Hyperkalaemia**

A causes metallic taste
B causes muscle weakness
C increases if sodium bicarbonate is given
D can be corrected by infusion of dextrose and insulin
E may cause no symptoms until cardiac arrest occurs

27.13   Adverse effects of diuretics include

A   magnesium deficiency
B   chronic hypovolaemia
C   hypoglycaemia
D   sexual impotence
E   gout

27.14   The following statements about osmotic diuretics are correct:

A   Osmotic diuretics act mainly in the collecting tubule where they prevent the reabsorption of water
B   Osmotic diuretics lower intracranial pressure primarily by inducing diuresis
C   Intravenous mannitol can lower intraocular pressure
D   An osmotic diuretic given to a patient with impaired renal function may cause pulmonary oedema
E   Exogenous urea can produce useful diuresis in patients with impaired renal function

27.15   Carbonic anhydrase inhibitors

A   cause alkaline urine to be formed
B   cause a metabolic acidosis
C   are drugs of choice for oedema
D   are useful for the prophylaxis of acute mountain sickness
E   cause intraocular pressure to rise

27.16   Cation-exchange resins

A   are as effective diuretics as are thiazides
B   are effective for the correction of hyperkalaemia
C   of sodium phase are preferred for patients with cardiac failure
D   of calcium phase should be avoided in patients with multiple myeloma
E   may be given rectally

27.17 When diuretic drugs are used

A their effectiveness can be monitored by body weight
B restriction of dietary salt to an unpleasant degree is usually unnecessary
C overdose is usually suggested by rising blood urea concentration
D to treat renal oedema, the combination of frusemide and metolazone is particularly effective
E to treat hepatic ascites, preliminary paracentesis is desirable

27.18 Oedema

A of cardiac origin may improve with bed rest
B of cardiac origin may improve with correction of anaemia
C of cardiac origin may improve if peripheral vascular resistance is reduced
D of hepatic origin should be treated with amiloride in preference to spironolactone
E may respond to frusemide by intravenous infusion when oral administration has been unsuccessful

27.19 Alkalinisation of the urine

A encourages the growth of *Esch. coli*
B reduces irritation in an inflamed urinary tract
C prevents urate stone formation
D increases urinary elimination of phenobarbitone
E increases urinary elimination of salicylate

27.20 Acidification of the urine

A increases urinary elimination of phencyclidine
B increases urinary elimination of amphetamine
C is produced by giving ascorbic acid
D discourages crystalluria with sulphonamides
E prevents cystine stone formation

27.21 **The kidney may be damaged by**

A gold
B amphotericin
C laxatives
D Worcestershire sauce
E aminoglycosides

27.22 **Substances that may precipitate in the urine and obstruct the urinary tract include**

A urate
B methotrexate
C sulphonamides
D calcium
E allopurinol

27.23 **Drugs that are eliminated almost exclusively by the kidney include**

A atenolol
B acyclovir
C propranolol
D rifampicin
E warfarin

27.24 **When prescribing a drug that is eliminated by the kidney for a patient with renal impairment**

A the initial dose should be lower than normal if there is hypoproteinaemia
B the creatinine clearance is a useful guide to dosage
C the normal maintenance dose may be given with the interval between doses being lengthened
D a reduced maintenance dose may be given with the interval between doses being unchanged
E the time to reach a steady state plasma concentration will be the same as in patients with normal renal function

27.25 **Drugs acceptable for patients with renal impairment include**

A dextroproxyphene
B methadone
C paracetamol
D phenytoin
E metformin

27.26 **Drugs acceptable for patients with renal impairment include**

A tetracycline
B nitrofurantoin
C captopril
D lithium
E temazepam

27.27 **The following statements about micturition are correct:**

A Phenoxybenzamine benefits incontinence due to spontaneous uninhibited contractions of the detrusor muscle
B Anticholinergic drugs alleviate obstructive symptoms in patients with prostatic hypertrophy by relaxing the proximal urethra
C Imipramine is effective for nocturnal and for daytime incontinence
D Androgens applied locally to the vagina may benefit urinary incontinence due to atrophy of the urethral epithelium in women
E Activation of α_1-adrenoceptors causes the smooth muscle of the internal urethral sphincter to contract

28 Blood I: Drugs and Haemostasis

28.1 **Vitamin K**

  A is necessary for the formation of Factor IX in the liver
  B requires bile for its absorption
  C restores reduced plasma prothrombin concentration to normal even in patients with severe liver damage
  D is widely distributed in plants
  E deficiency may occur as a result of small intestine resection

28.2 **The following statements are correct:**

  A Menadiol sodium phosphate may cause haemolytic anaemia
  B Phytomenadione is the most rapidly effective preparation of Vitamin K
  C It is best to use menadiol sodium phosphate for treating hypoprothrombinaemia in neonates
  D Hypoprothrombinaemia due to salicylate overdose resists treatment with Vitamin K
  E There is a danger of circulatory collapse if phytomenadione is given intravenously

28.3 Warfarin

A is the most generally satisfactory oral anticoagulant
B can be expected to achieve effective anticoagulant protection in 24–36 hours
C is monitored by regular determination of the prothrombin time expressed as a ratio
D should be avoided in early pregnancy because it inhibits the proper development of cartilage in the fetus
E is less likely to cause bleeding in the renal tract than into the joints

28.4 In anticoagulant treatment with warfarin

A 10–20mg/day is likely to be needed for effective maintenance therapy
B a prothrombin ratio of 2.0–2.5 is sufficient for prophylaxis of deep vein thrombosis
C the risk of bleeding is highest in patients with ischaemic cerebrovascular disease
D treatment of bleeding by Vitamin K takes several days to become effective even if the intravenous route is used
E the drug should on no account be stopped abruptly because of the risk of rebound thromboembolism

28.5 In patients on warfarin it is preferable (because of risk of drug interactions) to treat

A cardiac dysrhythmias with amiodarone rather than disopyramide
B convulsions with phenytoin rather than sodium valproate
C infections with metronidazole rather than a cephalosporin
D depression by tricyclic antidepressants
E patients requiring a β-adrenoceptor blocker with a water-soluble agent such as atenolol

28.6 Heparin

A was discovered by a medical student in the course of physiological research on blood clotting

B occurs in mast cells

C greatly enhances the activity of naturally occurring antithrombin III

D has a vasoconstrictor effect which limits its use in arterial embolism

E rarely requires the use of protamine sulphate to counter its effects

28.7 In treatment with heparin

A its effect can be measured by the prothrombin ratio as effectively as by the KCCT (kaolin cephalin clotting time)

B intravenous injection is required because it is precipitated by gastric acid

C all individuals respond to a standard dose to much the same extent

D thrombocytopenia occurs in less than 5% of patients

E osteoporosis tends to develop in patients on therapeutic doses for more than 4 months

28.8 Anticoagulant treatment in established venous thrombosis

A should be continued for as long as 6 months if there is any evidence of pulmonary embolus

B is unnecessary in the case of small distal thrombi

C is always preferred to streptokinase for thrombus in a large proximal vein

D is contraindicated in the presence of pulmonary hypertension

E is more effective than treatment with antiplatelet drugs

28.9　In the prevention of venous thrombosis

A　the use of oral anticoagulant has been limited by the effort needed to maintain control

B　there is no place for intermittent calf compression during surgery

C　heparin and dihydroergotamine should not be used together

D　low molecular weight dextran by i.v. injection may be useful

E　subcutaneous heparin is effective in as low a dose as 5,000 units 12-hourly

28.10　Long-term anticoagulant therapy

A　if well conducted carries no increased risk of haemorrhage

B　is indicated in cases of mitral stenosis with or without atrial fibrillation

C　prevents transient ischaemic attacks

D　should be used for most cases of intermittent claudication

E　is contraindicated in severe uncontrolled hypertension

28.11　In thrombolytic therapy

A　streptokinase is easier to use than urokinase since it is non-antigenic

B　both local and systemic infusion of a plasminogen activator may be useful

C　even the most susceptible thrombi take several days to disappear

D　recombinant tissue-type plasminogen activator may be superior to streptokinase

E　the complication of bleeding should be treated by tranexamic acid

28.12 **The following statements about blood platelet activity are correct:**

A Intact vascular endothelium does not attract platelets because of the high concentration of prostacyclin in the intima

B Thromboxane is derived mainly from platelets

C Dipyridamole reduces platelet activity by increasing cyclic AMP concentration

D There is no good evidence to suggest that aspirin may be of value in patients suffering from transient ischaemic attacks

E The beneficial role of fish consumption in the prevention of myocardial infarction is probably due to eicosapentaenoic acid

28.13 **The following statements about haemostatics are correct:**

A Adrenaline is only useful in epistaxis if given by injection

B The disadvantage of fibrin foam is that it is not absorbed in the body

C Tranexamic acid is of no value in the treatment of a haemophilic patient who has bled after tooth extraction

D Ethamsylate given systemically reduces bleeding in menorrhagia

E A freshly made solution of thrombin needs to be given by injection

29 Blood II: Iron, Vitamin B_{12} (cobalamin) and Folic Acid

29.1 Iron

A stores are as easily replenished by oral therapy as by injection

B in haemoglobin accounts for less than $\frac{1}{3}$ of total body iron

C released from destroyed erythrocytes is mostly excreted in the urine

D intake in the diet of an average Western man is 10–15 mg a day

E requirements in pregnancy are increased by over 2 mg daily

29.2 Absorption of iron

A is greater in an anaemic man than in a normal man

B is enhanced by ascorbic acid

C is more efficient if it is in ferric form

D is often reduced after partial gastrectomy

E takes place mostly in the upper small intestine

29.3 In iron deficiency

A the measurement of transferrin in the blood gives a good indication of the body's iron stores

B a high plasma ferritin is to be expected

C sore tongue is due to a reduction of iron-containing enzymes

D 25 mg of ferrous sulphate daily by mouth will produce a rise of 1% of haemoglobin per day

E it is important to give an initial loading dose of whatever iron preparation is used

29.4 In iron therapy

A iron dextran can be given only by intravenous infusion
B gastrointestinal upsets can be greatly influenced by the patient's anticipation of adverse effects
C tests for occult blood in the faeces are not generally interfered with
D intramuscular iron sorbitol causes the urine to turn black
E previously undetected folic acid deficiency is sometimes unmasked in the course of treatment

29.5 In acute iron poisoning

A symptoms are steadily progressive during the first 24 hours
B convulsions are to be expected within ½ hour of ingestion
C cardiovascular collapse is a feature
D an emetic is contraindicated
E raw egg and milk will help to bind iron until medical help is available

29.6 Desferrioxamine

A is excreted in the urine giving it a reddish colour
B is of little or no value in acute iron poisoning
C can cause goitre by binding cobalt in the gut
D is indicated in some haemolytic anaemias as well as in haemochromatosis
E is available as a topical eye formulation for ocular siderosis

29.7 Vitamin B$_{12}$

A stores in the body are enough to last for six weeks
B is normally absorbed in the ileum
C therapy by mouth is the first choice in pernicious anaemia
D is sensible trial therapy in undiagnosed anaemias
E deficiency would occur in wild rabbits if they did not eat their own faeces

29.8 Vitamin B$_{12}$ deficiency

A does not produce mental symptoms unless anaemia is present

B is most reliably diagnosed by a single stage Schilling test

C occurring in jejunal diverticular disease can be remedied by tetracycline

D is best treated by hydroxocobalamin because this is bound to plasma protein to a greater extent than cyanocobalamin

E may be complicated by hypokalaemia in severe cases responding briskly to treatment

29.9 Folic acid

A alone provides adequate treatment for some cases of pernicious anaemia

B is absorbed in the large intestine

C is only active when converted to tetrahydrofolic acid

D is not present in green vegetables other than spinach

E should be used routinely in pregnancy in a dose of about 300 μg a day

30 Respiratory System

30.1 Cough

A that is due to a cause above the larynx often responds to a demulcent

B that is due to a cause below the larynx often responds to water aerosol and benzoin inhalation

C is reduced by opioids

D is improved by antihistamines through block of histamine H_1-receptors

E is little affected by psychogenic factors

30.2 The following statements about mucus and mucolytics are correct:

A Bromhexine assists mucus clearance by causing bronchodilation

B Acetylcysteine increases sputum viscosity

C Iodide stimulates production of thin bronchial secretion by direct action on secretory cells

D Sputum viscosity may be lowered by rehydrating a patient

E Mucolytics cause gastrointestinal symptoms

30.3 The following statements about respiratory stimulation are correct:

A Respiratory stimulation is usually necesary in the management of an acute asthmatic attack

B Respiratory stimulation may be useful in the management of acute ventilatory failure with hypercapnia due to exacerbation of chronic lung disease

C Doxapram has a larger margin between therapeutic and toxic doses than do other respiratory stimulants

D Patients with epilepsy may safely be given respiratory stimulants

E Aminophylline can provide useful respiratory stimulation for apnoeic premature infants

30.4 Oxygen

A comprises 21% of atmospheric air

B in arterial blood at a partial pressure of 6.7 kPa is adequate to maintain tissue oxygenation in chronically hypoxic patients

C should not be used in high concentration (60%) even for short periods for patients with pulmonary embolism lest the hypoxic drive for respiration be removed

D **must normally be used in concentrations exceeding 28% to provide adequate therapy for patients with infective exacerbations of chronic obstructive lung disease**

E as continuous long-term (domiciliary) therapy improves survival in patients with severe persistent hypoxia and cor pulmonale due to chronic bronchitis and emphysema

30.5 Histamine

A acts principally as a systemic hormone

B causes capillaries to dilate

C inhibits gastric secretion

D causes bronchial muscle to relax

E causes itch

30.6 **Some or all of the consequences of histamine release in the body can be opposed or prevented by**

A adrenaline
B cimetidine
C astemizole
D prednisolone
E sodium cromoglycate

30.7 **Some histamine H$_1$-receptor antagonists are used**

A as hypnotics
B to treat Parkinson's disease
C as antitussives
D to treat acute urticaria
E to treat peptic ulcer

30.8 **The following statements about histamine H$_1$-receptor antagonists are correct:**

A Histamine H$_1$-receptor antagonists generally are competitive inhibitors of the action of histamine
B At therapeutic doses astemizole exhibits unsurmountable antagonism of the action of histamine
C Histamine H$_1$-receptor antagonists are more effective if used before histamine has been liberated
D Terfenadine does not potentiate the sedative effects of alcohol
E Promethazine is free from sedative effects

30.9 The following statements about allergic states are correct:

A In hay fever, rebound swelling of the nasal mucous membrane occurs when topical vasoconstrictor medication is stopped

B In severe angioneurotic oedema, s.c. adrenaline provides quickest relief

C In cold urticaria combined histamine H_1- and H_2-receptor antagonism may be needed fully to block the vascular effects

D Hereditary angioedema does not respond to antihistamines and should be treated with fresh frozen plasma

E Non-urticarial drug eruptions may be made worse by H_1-antihistamines

30.10 In asthma

A the principal inflammatory bronchoconstrictor mediator is histamine

B early in an attack hyperventilation maintains the PaO_2 and keeps the $PaCO_2$ low

C immediate reactions to inhaled allergens occur in non-atopic persons

D some patients exhibit wheeze and breathlessness that is not attributable to any known allergen

E some patients develop wheeze that regularly follows within a few minutes of exercise

30.11 In asthma

A identification of an antigen may be aided by testing the patient's blood

B anxiety is best alleviated by propranolol

C β-adrenoceptor agonists are preferred therapy

D bronchial mucosal vasoconstriction with an adrenaline spray is useful

E drugs with antimuscarinic action may be beneficial

30.12 Sodium cromoglycate

A is effective in the management of an acute attack of asthma
B is of no use in asthmatic children
C is most effective when given by the oral route
D does not interfere with hyposensitisation procedures
E causes drowsiness

30.13 Theophylline

A t½ is increased in patients with severe cardiopulmonary disease
B at a plasma concentration of 40 mg/l achieves optimum bronchodilation with fewest adverse effects
C in overdose causes cardiac dysrhythmia
D by suppository at night is effective for 'morning dippers'
E should be given in reduced dose by the intravenous route for an acute asthmatic attack if the patient has received the drug in the previous 24 h

30.14 The following statements about the treatment of asthma are correct:

A Failure to respond to a metered dose aerosol is often due to improper technique of its use
B Ipratropium by metered dose aerosol may benefit elderly intrinsic asthmatics
C Reduced hypothalamic-pituitary-adrenal responsiveness is a significant problem with the use of inhaled corticosteroids
D Inhaled corticosteroid may cause oropharyngeal candidiasis
E Adrenal suppression with oral corticosteroid may be minimised by giving a single evening dose

30.15 In status asthmaticus

A salbutamol may be given by nebulised aerosol
B ipratropium may be given by nebulised aerosol
C hydrocortisone is preferred to prednisolone for initial therapy
D humidified oxygen should be given
E morphine provides useful sedation

31 Gastrointestinal System I: Control of Gastric Secretion and Mucosal Resistance: Peptic Ulcer

31.1 Histamine H$_2$-receptor antagonists

A increase the healing rate of peptic ulcers
B do not prevent relapse of peptic ulcers
C do not benefit reflux oesophagitis
D do not relieve symptoms if there is early gastric cancer
E lose therapeutic efficacy if an antacid is used at the same time

31.2 Cimetidine

A inhibits hepatic metabolism of other drugs
B inhibits gastric secretion stimulated by caffeine
C has been shown to be beneficial in patients bleeding as a result of Mallory-Weiss syndrome
D controls diarrhoea in the Zollinger Ellison syndrome
E may cause gynaecomastia

31.3 In the treatment of peptic ulcer the following statements are correct:

A Ranitidine reduces gastric acid less effectively than does cimetidine
B Pirenzepine reduces gastric acid through its anticholinergic action
C Some prostaglandin analogues have a mucosal protective action
D Proton pump inhibitors such as omeprazole produce profound and prolonged inhibition of gastric acid secretion
E Antacids do not affect the acid-base balance of the body

31.4   The following statements about antacids are correct:

A   Metabolic alkalosis is more likely to occur with sodium bicarbonate than with other antacids

B   Magnesium salts cause diarrhoea

C   Calcium-containing antacids should be avoided since they may produce renal damage ·

D   Aluminium hydroxide is the antacid of choice for patients in renal failure

E   All antacids are likely to produce oedema in patients with cardiac disease

31.5   The following drugs enhance peptic ulcer healing by a local/topical effect:

A   Dimethicone

B   Bismuth chelate

C   Bran

D   Sucralfate

E   Carbenoxolone

32 Gastrointestinal System II: Drugs for Vomiting, Constipation and Diarrhoea

32.1 The vomiting centre and its chemoreceptor trigger zone contain

A adrenoceptors
B acetylcholine receptors
C dopamine receptors
D histamine H_1-receptors
E serotonin (5HT) receptors

32.2 Drugs which may benefit motion sickness include

A hyoscine
B cyclizine
C promethazine
D cimetidine
E dimenhydrinate

32.3 Drugs which may benefit nausea and vomiting from any cause include

A domperidone
B chlorpromazine
C nabilone
D prochlorperazine
E metoclopramide

32.4 Metoclopramide

A is if no value in migraine
B acts centrally by blocking dopamine receptors in the chemoreceptor trigger zone (CTZ)
C acts on smooth muscle in the gut
D is less likely to cause extrapyramidal dystonic reactions than is domperidone
E may cause gynaecomastia

32.5 In motion sickness

A prevention is easier than cure
B nabilone is often used
C the use of cyclizine is limited by its frequent side effects
D both meclozine and promethazine may cause sleepiness
E hyoscine is preferred for prolonged use

32.6 The following statements are correct:

A Phenothiazines are useful in the treatment of reflux oesophagitis
B Hiccup may respond to prochlorperazine
C Peppermint may be useful in the irritable bowel syndrome
D Chlorophyll stimulates appetite as effectively as gentian
E Vertigo may be benefited by sedation and an antiemetic

32.7 The following statements about bulk purgatives are correct:

A They act by reducing the volume and raising the viscosity of bowel contents

B Bran may cause intestinal obstruction if taken with too little water

C Methylcellulose is used in the control of colostomies

D Saline purgatives should be used with special care in patients with renal failure

E In a patient with laxative dependence bulk purgatives are more likely to cause protein-losing enteropathy than are stimulant purgatives

32.8 The following statements are correct:

A Lactulose is an osmotic purgative

B Lactulose benefits hepatic encephalopathy by acid fermentation in the colon

C Bran enters the colon intact

D One gram of bran can hold 23 grams of water

E Docusate sodium softens hard faeces

32.9 The following statements about stimulant purgatives are correct:

A They are used to clear the colon for radiological examination

B Bisacodyl suppositories are useful in geriatric patients

C Excessive use does not damage the colon

D Phenolphthalein turns alkaline urine red

E During pregnancy senna is preferred to castor oil

32.10 Liquid paraffin

A has an unpleasant taste
B allows more water to remain in the bowel, as does docusate sodium
C if taken at night over long periods carries a risk of lipoid pneumonia
D is chemically inert
E if used long term is associated with a slightly increased risk of gastrointestinal cancer

32.11 Oral rehydration therapy of acute diarrhoea

A is effectively achieved by a solution containing glucose, sodium, chloride, potassium and bicarbonate
B alone is sufficient to treat most episodes of watery diarrhoea
C should be routinely supplemented by antimicrobial agents in cases of travellers' diarrhoea
D is not well achieved by commercial soft drinks because of their low sodium content
E should always be accompanied by an antimotility drug in controlling severe diarrhoea in young children

32.12 In the treatment of diarrhoea

A kaolin directly increases the viscosity of gut contents
B drugs of the opium group reduce peristalsis
C naloxone is ineffective against respiratory depression due to overdose of diphenoxylate
D anticholinergic drugs are valueless
E occurring in international travellers codeine phosphate is likely to provide socially useful reduction in frequency of stools

32.13 Treatment of a severe attack of ulcerative colitis includes

A a broad spectrum antibiotic
B at least three litres of fluid and electrolytes daily
C intravenous prednisolone
D hydrocortisone by intrarectal drip
E large doses of azathioprine

32.14 Sulphasalazine

A is a prodrug that is activated in the colon
B is preferable to metronidazole in the management of perianal Crohn's disease
C can be usefully substituted by mesalazine (5-aminosalicylic acid) if it is not well tolerated
D causes side effects which are commoner in genetically slow acetylators
E causes reversible infertility in men

33 Gastrointestinal System III: Liver and Biliary Tract

33.1 Drug-induced hepatic injury due to

A paracetamol is not dose dependent

B methotrexate can be minimised by using small doses over a long period

C an androgen is more likely to occur in the case of a drug that is active only when injected

D chlorpromazine is cholestatic

E rifampicin only occurs after several months of treatment

33.2 In a patient with cirrhosis of the liver

A drugs normally subject to hepatic first pass metabolism have a low systemic availability

B morphine is safe

C diuretics need to be used with particular care

D MAO inhibitors are less hazardous than tricyclic antidepressants

E antimicrobials normally eliminated by the kidney are safe

33.3 In a patient with gallstones

A chenodeoxycholic acid can be expected to dissolve calcified stones provided that they are very small

B drug treatment is likely to require 24 months to be effective

C ursodeoxycholic acid is less likely to cause diarrhoea than chenodeoxycholic acid

D a terpene mixture (Rowachol) may be helpful if stones are present in the common bile duct

E cholestyramine is only indicated to relieve pruritus if bile-duct obstruction is complete

34 Endocrinology I: Adrenal Cortex, Corticotrophin, Corticosteroids and Antagonists

34.1 **The naturally occurring physiologically important secretions of the adrenal cortex include**

A cortisone
B hydrocortisone
C prednisolone
D aldosterone
E androgens

34.2 **The following statements about natural corticotrophin are correct:**

A It is a polypeptide consisting of 39 aminoacids
B Its biological activity resides in the first 24 aminoacids
C Its immunological antigenic activity resides in the final 15 aminoacids
D It has a plasma t½ of 3 h
E The response of the adrenal cortex to a rise in plasma corticotrophin begins after 30 minutes

34.3 **Natural corticotrophin**

A is active when taken by mouth
B is the major controlling factor in hydrocortisone production by the adrenal cortex
C is the major controlling factor in aldosterone production by the adrenal cortex
D is a preferred treatment for Addison's disease (primary adrenocortical insufficiency)
E is a preferred treatment for secondary adrenocortical insufficiency (hypopituitarism)

34.4 Tetracosactrin

A   is a synthetic polypeptide
B   has an aminoacid structure identical with natural corticotrophin
C   is more liable to induce immunological adverse reactions (allergy) than is corticotrophin obtained from animals
D   has a plasma t½ much longer than natural corticotrophin
E   is active when taken by mouth

34.5 Corticoliberin (corticotrophin-releasing hormone, CRH)

A   is secreted by the hypothalamus in response to changing plasma concentrations of hydrocortisone
B   secretion is unaffected by environmental stress
C   secretion is unaffected by prednisolone administered for anti-inflammatory or immunosuppressive purposes
D   production is suppressed less during therapy with corticotrophin than with synthetic corticosteroids
E   is released in response to insulin hypoglycaemia and thus can be used to test the integrity of the hypothalamic/ pituitary/adrenal axis

34.6 In choosing between corticotrophin and a synthetic corticosteroid for therapy of asthma, account should be taken of the following:

A   Muscle wasting and osteoporosis are more likely with corticotrophin
B   Acne and hypertension are more likely with corticotrophin
C   Sudden withdrawal of therapy and intercurrent illness are less hazardous with corticotrophin
D   Adrenocortical atrophy is more prominent with synthetic corticosteroids
E   Growth suppression in children is a serious problem with corticotrophin

34.7 The following corticosteroids are prodrugs:

A Hydrocortisone
B Cortisone
C Prednisone
D Prednisolone
E Methylprednisolone

34.8 The following statements about adrenocortical steroids are correct:

A The actions of adrenocortical steroids are classified as mineralocorticoid and glucocorticoid
B Mineralocorticoid actions principally enhance sodium excretion and potassium retention
C Glucocorticoid actions principally affect metabolism of carbohydrate, protein and fat
D Glucocorticoid actions include suppression of inflammation and of immune responses
E Systemic administration of substantial doses induces suppression of the hypothalamic-pituitary-adrenocortical system via a feedback mechanism

34.9 The following corticosteroids have largely or exclusively glucocorticoid actions:

A Dexamethasone
B Hydrocortisone
C Fludrocortisone
D Prednisolone
E Cortisone

34.10 **An adrenal cortex suppressed by administration of a high therapeutic dose of adrenocortical steroid**

A continues to secrete androgen
B continues to secrete aldosterone
C will recover independently of hypothalamic-pituitary function
D puts the patient at hazard due to intercurrent disease
E puts patients at hazard if they lose their tablets

34.11 **The following statements about the quantitative aspects of adrenocortical steroid function and therapy are correct:**

A The normal daily secretion of hydrocortisone is 10 to 30 mg which is equivalent to 4 to 6 mg prednisolone for glucocorticoid effect
B Twenty mg prednisolone administered daily will induce substantial suppression of the adrenal cortex
C High doses (pharmacotherapy) of corticosteroid induce clinically important suppression of the hypothalamic-pituitary-adrenocortical axis in less than one week
D Recovery of hypothalamic-pituitary-adrenocortical function is complete one week after withdrawal of a suppressive dose of corticosteroid
E Serious adverse effects of long term pharmacotherapy are in general unlikely if the daily dose of corticosteroid is less than 15 mg prednisolone or its equivalent

34.12 **Adrenocortical steroids are used**

A as replacement therapy in adrenocortical insufficiency
B to suppress bacterial inflammation and antibody formation in shock
C in neonatal respiratory distress syndrome
D to suppress immunological inflammation
E to suppress the rejection of transplanted organs

34.13 **The following choices of corticosteroid are appropriate:**

A Prednisone for replacement therapy
B Beclomethasone for inhalation in asthma
C Cortisone for immunosuppression
D Prednisolone for anti-inflammation
E Dexamethasone for reduction of intracranial pressure

34.14 **The following statements about adrenocortical steroid therapy are correct:**

A Atrophy of the adrenal cortex in long-term treatment is due to a direct effect on the hypothalamus
B There are no differences in the incidence of adverse effects with the principal corticosteroids
C Therapy should be stopped immediately an adverse effect appears
D Serious systemic adverse effects of topical (eg to skin) therapy are less likely with fluorinated than with non-fluorinated corticosteroids
E Sometimes a corticosteroid is given with the intention of suppressing (inhibiting) the hypothalamic-pituitary-adrenal axis

34.15 **Replacement therapy with corticosteroid**

A is best conducted with hydrocortisone because it has both mineralocorticoid and glucocorticoid effects
B is devised to mimic the pattern of natural hormone secretion during day and night
C is conducted at higher doses than pharmacotherapy
D may require added salt for optimal effect
E usually includes a small dose of fludrocortisone

34.16 **In long-term corticosteroid pharmacotherapy for anti-inflammatory effect**

A beclomethasone is especially useful as it is not absorbed from the lung

B triamcinolone is liable to cause muscle wasting

C prednisolone is preferable to hydrocortisone because prednisolone has selective glucocorticoid actions

D cortisone is the drug of choice in patients with liver damage

E an injection of corticotrophin should be given regularly to prevent cortical atrophy

34.17 **The following statements about synthetic corticosteroids are correct:**

A They have a plasma t½ of 1–3 h

B Their t½ is unaffected by liver disease or hepatic enzyme induction

C Alterations to plasma protein binding due to disease or other drugs may cause misleading results in laboratory tests eg for Cushing's syndrome

D Serious adverse effects such as osteoporosis may occur with as few as two doses

E In long term therapy the minimum effective dose should be used

34.18 **Intermittent or alternate-day dosage with adrenocortical steroids**

A minimises hypothalamic-pituitary-adrenocortical suppression

B may be useful in replacement therapy for adrenocortical insufficiency

C is worth trying when immunosuppression is the objective

D is of particular value in rheumatoid arthritis

E minimises the risk of growth suppression in children

34.19 Long-term adrenocortical steroid therapy carries an extra risk of adverse effects in patients giving a history of

A mental disorder
B peptic ulcer
C hypertension
D tuberculosis
E diabetes mellitus

34.20 Active immunisation of patients taking long-term corticosteroid pharmacotherapy (for suppression of inflammation or immune responses)

A should never be attempted in children
B is hazardous with a killed vaccine
C is hazardous with a live vaccine
D is hazardous with a toxoid vaccine
E may be ineffective if the dose of corticosteroid is high

34.21 If a patient on long-term corticosteroid therapy (whether for replacement or pharmacotherapy) develops an intercurrent illness, he should

A omit the next dose
B inform his doctor
C take large doses of oral potassium
D save a specimen of urine for the doctor to test
E post his 'steroid card' to the Department of Health and Social Security

34.22 Precautions to be taken during high dose long-term corticosteroid pharmacotherapy include

A regular weighing
B regular blood pressure measurement
C a regular urine test for sugar
D carrying a special card recording the details of treatment
E paying serious attention to any illness, however slight

34.23 **Adverse effects of long-term corticosteroid pharmacotherapy include**

A osteoporosis
B hypertension
C muscle wasting
D deficient blood coagulation
E easy bruising

34.24 **A patient who has taken corticosteroid for a long time may develop**

A psychotic reactions
B increased growth in children
C menstrual disorders
D major skin damage after quite minor injury
E raised intracranial pressure

34.25 **Long-term corticosteroid pharmacotherapy may lead to**

A acromegaly
B serious delayed tissue healing after surgery
C increased severity of infections
D masking of infections, which may produce atypical clinical features
E activation of dormant infections

34.26 **Prolonged corticosteroid pharmacotherapy causes**

A oedema
B insomnia
C glaucoma
D diabetes mellitus
E acne

34.27 The following statements about withdrawing adrenocorticosteroid pharmacotherapy that has lasted for many weeks are correct:

A The patient is at risk of acute adrenal insufficiency because the adrenal cortex has atrophied

B The longer the duration of therapy, the slower must be the withdrawal

C Corticotrophin should be given to hasten recovery of the adrenal cortex

D If a patient cannot take the dose orally there should be no hesitation in using an injectable (i.m.) preparation

E If a patient requires surgery during, or even one year after withdrawal, a careful scheme of added corticosteroid administration is required

34.28 In pregnancy

A corticosteroid pharmacotherapy is not suspected of causing fetal injury

B fluorinated corticosteroids carry teratogenic hazard, even if applied to the skin

C hypoadrenal patients on replacement therapy require no special management

D labour is managed like major surgery

E the administration of corticosteroid pharmacotherapy to the mother does not affect the newborn child

34.29 The following statements about adrenocortical hormone synthesis and function are correct:

A Spironolactone is a competitive antagonist of aldosterone

B Metyrapone blocks corticosteroid receptors

C Metyrapone interferes with the enzymic synthesis of hydrocortisone

D Metyrapone can be used as a test for the capacity of the hypothalamic-pituitary axis to produce corticotrophin

E Trilostane interferes with enzymic synthesis of hydrocortisone and of aldosterone

35 Endocrinology II: Diabetes Mellitus: Insulin, Oral Hypoglycaemics

35.1 Insulin

A was discovered in Canada
B output by the pancreas is 30–40 units daily
C no longer has to be standardised biologically to provide worldwide uniformity
D is stored in the liver
E is a polypeptide

35.2 Insulin causes

A reduction of hepatic output of glucose
B reduction of protein synthesis
C enhanced transit of potassium into cells
D increased glucose uptake in peripheral tissues
E down regulation of insulin receptors when its concentration is high, a factor in the insulin resistance of obese diabetics

35.3 When insulin is injected

A about half the dose can be recovered from the urine
B its plasma t½ is about 10 minutes
C and hypoglycaemia results, corticotrophin is released from the pituitary
D the intravenous route is preferred in severe ketoacidosis
E subcutaneous lipoatrophy is unknown nowadays

35.4   The following statements about insulin preparations are correct:

A   Insulin Zinc Suspension acts longer in its amorphous form than in its crystalline form

B   The chief reason for using human insulin is reduced immunogenicity

C   New diabetics requiring insulin should be started on HP (highly purified) or MC (monocomponent) insulin of animal or human origin

D   Neutral (soluble) insulin should not be mixed in the syringe with Insulin Zinc Suspensions

E   A single standard strength of insulin preparations (100 IU per ml) is replacing the wide range of strengths previously standard

35.5   Soluble insulin

A   is more likely to cause local discomfort in a formulation at pH3 than at pH7

B   if infused in a saline drip is subject to substantial loss as a result of binding to the tubing

C   has a peak action at 30–60 minutes when given intravenously

D   is particularly useful for balancing patients who have heavy glycosuria before breakfast

E   is the only preparation suitable for intravenous use

35.6   A hypoglycaemic attack

A   should always be treated by sugar (sucrose or glucose) in the first instance

B   which does not respond to glucose within thirty minutes suggests that dexamethasone may be useful as the patient may have cerebral oedema

C   is never fatal

D   should only be treated by glucagon injections if there has been no response one hour after intravenous glucose

E   is less likely to occur in patients treated with insulin than in those on sulphonylureas

**35.7   The following statements about oral hypoglycaemic drugs
are correct:**

A   Biguanides are effective even in the absence of insulin
B   Sulphonylureas act by stimulating the β-islet cells of the
pancreas
C   Chlorpropamide is safer than tolbutamide in patients with
poor renal function
D   Lactic acidosis limits the use of biguanides
E   Glibenclamide has the disadvantage of having to be taken
three times a day

35.8   In the treatment of diabetes it is generally accepted that

A   patients should reduce their insulin dosage if they
develop fever
B   some drugs may interfere with both blood and urine
glucose estimations
C   it is best to control maturity onset diabetes by weight
reduction alone
D   once a patient has been stabilised on an oral
hypoglycaemic drug, close supervision is no longer
needed
E   good control of blood sugar reduces the incidence of
neuropathy

35.9   In a pregnant diabetic patient

A   oral hypoglycaemic agents are preferable to insulin
B   insulin requirements fall during lactation
C   the renal threshold for glucose rises in the third trimester
D   maternal hyperglycaemia leads to fetal islet cell
hyperplasia
E   all treatment should be stopped during labour

35.10 Drugs which can disturb the control of a diabetic patient include

A monoamine oxidase inhibitors
B sulphonamides
C aspirin
D thiazide diuretics
E oral contraceptives

35.11 In diabetic ketoacidosis

A it is sometimes difficult to decide whether to use insulin or an oral hypoglycaemic drug
B hypomagnesaemia is a problem as often as hypokalaemia
C insulin is best given by continuous low-dose infusion
D treatment with bicarbonate is not useful and may even be harmful
E stringent precautions against septicaemia are necessary

35.12 In a diabetic undergoing major surgery

A a high blood glucose concentration, even for a short time, is particularly dangerous
B insulin is indicated even if there has been previous good control by oral hypoglycaemic drugs
C insulin requirements are likely to be higher as a result of operation
D glucose by mouth should be given one hour preoperatively
E ketoacidosis should be controlled, if possible, in all cases before operation, even in a surgical emergency

36 Endocrinology III: Thyroid Hormones: Antithyroid Drugs

36.1 Thyroid hormone

A consists of T4 and T3
B exerts its effect chiefly through T3 to which T4 is converted
C is 99.9% bound to plasma protein
D acts on specific receptors on target organ cells
E is stored in the gland as thyroglobulin

36.2 The following statements about thyroid function are correct:

A Tests involving measurement of radioiodine uptake are now hardly ever used
B Thyrotrophin-releasing hormone (TRH) is used to determine whether or not hypothyroidism is secondary to pituitary or hypothalamic disease
C TSH (thyrotrophin) can be measured in the blood
D Exophthalmos is now known to be directly due to increased secretion of thyroid hormone
E The goitre which sometimes occurs during therapy with antithyroid drugs is due to increased formation of TSH

36.3 Treatment with thyroxine

A can reduce the size of puberty goitre
B for hypothyroidism in an old patient should start in a dosage of 1 mg daily
C need only be continued in a cretin until the age of five years
D is of great value in the management of simple obesity
E in an adult is difficult because the dosage needs to be changed so frequently

36.4 **The following statements about thyroid hormone treatment are correct:**

A Liothyronine finds its main use in myxoedema coma

B A dose of liothyronine gives maximum effect in about 24 h and passes off over a week

C A dose of thyroxine gives a maximum effect in about 10 days and passes off over 2 to 3 weeks

D Overtreatment causes atrial fibrillation in patients over 60 years

E Overtreatment causes exophthalmos

36.5 **Iodine or iodide**

A is present in most radiographic contrast media

B is an effective antiseptic

C given preoperatively makes thyroidectomy easier and safer

D in very small amounts are useful in cough medicines

E can cause hyperthyroidism

36.6 **The following statements about thiourea derivatives are correct:**

A They inhibit the coupling of iodotyrosine to form T4 and T3

B They are goitrogenic

C They are not useful in a thyroid crisis (storm)

D Carbimazole cannot be expected to cause any clinical improvement in less than a month

E They have no measurable effect on the ankle reflex time

36.7 **When drug therapy is used to control thyroid function**

A propranolol quickly relieves symptoms in hyperthyroidism

B propranolol is not useful if radioiodine is being used

C β-adrenoceptor blockade is especially useful in thyrotoxic heart failure

D guanethidine eyedrops may improve lid retraction

E treatment should not be stopped while a thyroid bruit persists

36.8 The following statements about the use of radioiodine are correct:

A All hyperthyroid patients treated with radioiodine are likely to need treatment for hypothyroidism eventually

B The effect is maximal in 3 weeks

C Women of child-bearing age should be advised not to get pregnant for a few months after treatment

D It has been shown that there is no increased risk of leukaemia even after the high doses needed for treatment of thyroid carcinoma

E Radioiodine treatment is preferable to surgery if there is obstruction of neck veins

37 Endocrinology IV: Hypothalamic and Pituitary Hormones: Sex Hormones, Contraception, Uterus

37.1 Among the anterior pituitary hormones

A somatrem (methionyl human growth hormone) stimulates cell growth both for number and size

B human chorionic gonadotrophin (HCG) cannot be recovered from the urine of pregnant women

C prolactin is secreted only by women

D the plasma half-life of corticotrophin is 10 minutes

E neither HCG nor LH are of value in cryptorchidism

37.2 In infertility

A in a hypopituitary female, treatment with FSH alone can be expected to result in a sustained pregnancy

B of non-hypopituitary anovular origin, blockade of hypothalamic oestrogen receptors may result in pregnancy

C clomiphene treatment carries an increased risk of multiple pregnancy

D tamoxifen has a part to play in the treatment of both female and male infertility

E testosterone is the hormone of choice in the treatment of male infertility

37.3 Vasopressin

A increases water reabsorption in the distal renal tubule

B secretion is stimulated by nicotine

C deficiency may occur in hypopituitarism

D is a useful drug to raise the blood pressure

E should not be used to control bleeding from oesophageal varices if there is evidence of myocardial ischaemia

37.4   In diabetes insipidus

A   thiazide diuretics sometimes have an antidiuretic effect
B   glibenclamide may produce clinical improvement
C   clofibrate is contraindicated
D   dilutional hyponatraemia may occur
E   desmopressin is the treatment of choice

37.5   The syndrome of inappropriate antidiuretic hormone secretion (SIADH)

A   is caused only by oat-cell lung cancer
B   is subject to the normal homeostatic mechanisms
C   may need treatment with infusion of hypertonic saline in acute cases
D   may be usefully treated by demeclocycline
E   is unaffected by chemotherapy to the causal tumour

37.6   Oxytocin

A   treatment, if prolonged, carries a risk of severe water intoxication
B   can be used to enhance milk ejection from the breast
C   obtained from the posterior pituitary gland is safer than the synthetic product (Syntocinon)
D   treatment mimics normal uterine activity in labour
E   given by the buccal route carries a lesser risk of uterine rupture than if the intravenous route is used

37.7   Testosterone

A   is necessary for spermatogenesis as well as for growth of the sexual apparatus
B   is preferable to methyltestosterone in the control of itching in a jaundiced patient
C   is antagonised by cyproterone
D   may be beneficial in fibrocystic disease of the breast
E   slows the rate of closure of epiphyses of bone

37.8 Cyproterone

A has an affinity for androgen receptors both on the hypothalamus and on target organs
B is a derivative of progesterone
C causes irreversible reduction of spermatogenesis in males
D is used in female hirsutism
E exacerbates acne

37.9 When treated with a protein anabolic agent

A adult males run a substantial risk of hypermasculinisation
B patients with advanced malignant disease may derive benefit
C the itching of jaundice may lessen
D men with osteoporosis can be expected to improve
E patients with bone metastases from breast cancer can expect to avoid the complication of hypercalcaemia

37.10 The following statements about oestrogens are correct:

A Natural oestrogens have several advantages over synthetic oestrogens
B Bleeding may occur as a result of endometrial infarcts even though oestrogen levels are high
C The use of stilboestrol is confined to the treatment of oestrogen-dependent breast or prostate cancers
D The secretion of parathormone is depressed when oestrogens are used to treat osteoporosis
E Patients with senile vaginitis using oestrogen pessaries do not develop systemic effects of treatment

37.11 In oestrogen replacement therapy

A 'unopposed' treatment (ie without added progestogen) causes an increased risk of endometrial carcinoma
B continuous treatment is preferable to interrupted courses
C the minimal effective dose should be given
D cyclical use is essential in hysterectomised women
E for menopausal symptoms, treatment should on no account be stopped under three years

37.12 Oestrogen treatment

A is indicated in large doses for prostatic carcinoma
B may control recurrent epistaxis
C may result in painful gynaecomastia in men
D may worsen diabetes
E inhibits lactation by the same mechanism that bromocriptine does

37.13 The following statements about progesterone or synthetic progestogens are correct:

A Progesterone is necessary for implantation of the ovum
B Treatment is clearly beneficial in habitual abortion even if occurrence of true progesterone deficiency cannot be established
C Administration of a synthetic progestogen to the mother can virilise a female fetus
D A slow release progestogen formulation can be given via an intrauterine contraceptive device for local endometrial effect
E Danazol, though derived from a progestogen, has a mix of antiprogestogen and androgen actions

37.14 In the control of conception

A gonadorelin (LH/FSHRH), used continuously, suppresses spermatogenesis by down regulation of its receptors
B pheromones are likely to be useful in the near future
C vaginal preparations such as nonoxinol are highly reliable if properly used
D inactivation of pituitary gonadotrophins by immunological techniques is being developed
E postcoital oestrogen/progestogen treatment can only be effective within an hour of coitus

37.15 The effects of oral contraception with a mixture of oestrogen and progestogen include

A decreased viscosity of cervical mucus
B a substantial risk of harming an undiagnosed pregnancy
C decreased glucose tolerance
D liability to migraine
E a decreased risk of developing thromboembolism

37.16 Users of oral oestrogen/progestogen contraceptives in Britain

A have a higher death rate than those using an intrauterine device in all age groups
B are more likely to develop cardiovascular complications if they smoke
C have a chance of about 1 in 300 of becoming pregnant
D are not at increased risk for the development of gallbladder disease
E have more ectopic gestations than do vaginal diaphragm users

37.17 In the treatment of menstruation and its disorders

A the premenstrual tension syndrome is now generally agreed to be well controlled by bromocriptine
B dysmenorrhoea is usefully treated by inhibitors of prostaglandin synthesis
C menstruation can be advanced by giving norethisterone
D menorrhagia may be reduced by norethisterone
E all cases of amenorrhoea should be treated by cyclical hormone replacement therapy

37.18 **The following statements about ergot derivatives are correct:**

A Ergometrine and oxytocin have identical actions on the uterus

B Bromocriptine was produced for its prolactin-inhibiting effect

C Ergotamine is an α-adrenoceptor agonist

D Co-dergocrine (Hydergine) can have modest beneficial effect on impaired mental function in the aged

E Ergometrine can cause severe hypertension

37.19 **Prostaglandins**

A are anti-inflammatory agents

B occur only in the seminal vesicles and the central nervous system

C may cause uterine contraction or relaxation according to circumstances

D cannot yet be synthesised

E are used to induce abortion

38 Malignant Disease: Cytotoxic Chemotherapy: Immunosuppression

38.1 **In the chemotherapy of malignant disease the following statements are historically correct:**

A The first attempt to control cancer by means other than surgery was not made until the end of the nineteenth century

B Observation that oophorectomy prolonged lactation in cows led to the suggestion that some cases of breast cancer are dependent on ovarian function

C The unreliability of plasma acid phosphatase concentration as a marker of activity held up the development of oestrogen treatment for prostatic cancer for several years

D Depression of haemopoiesis by sulphur mustards (the precursors of nitrogen mustards) was observed when they were used as chemical weapons in the 1914–18 war

E Nitrogen mustards had to be tested first on man since no satisfactory animal model was available

38.2 **Success of chemotherapy in malignant disease depends on**

A a good immune response to treatment

B the size of the tumour

C the number of cells dividing at any one time

D the endocrine environment of the malignant cell

E the rate of recovery of normal tissues from the effects of treatment

38.3 Cancer cells

A have less differentiated morphology than the tissue of origin

B divide more rapidly than the cells in any normal organ

C have a longer survival time if a large number are initially present

D are generally most sensitive to drugs when they are in a resting phase

E are not subject to the normal feedback mechanism which restricts cell multiplication

38.4 Factors which tend to make an ageing cancer less susceptible to drugs include

A increased capacity for metastasis

B increased cell cycle (division) time

C failure of normal marrow to recover quickly from the effects of cytotoxic agents

D exponential shortening of volume-doubling time

E overcrowding of cells, denying access to drugs

38.5 The following statements on principles of chemotherapy in cancer are correct:

A A given dose of drug kills a constant *number* of cells, however many are present

B Selectivity of drugs for cancer cells is less in lymphoma than in other tumours

C One of the advantages of combined therapy is that it can reduce toxicity to bone marrow

D Inadequate initial therapy is the usual reason for failure to control choriocarcinoma

E Resistance to drugs occurs as a result of factors which are quite dissimilar from those involved in the development of bacterial resistance

38.6 **In planning intermittent combination therapy**

A vincristine is used to synchronise active cell cycles

B most regimens have been devised on a basis of commonsense empiricism

C intervals between courses of drugs should be at least two months

D the aim of MVPP (mustine, vinblastine, procarbazine, prednisolone) is total cell kill

E overlap of toxicities between the drugs chosen is of little importance

38.7 **Adverse effects of anticancer drugs include**

A depression of both antibody and cell mediated immunity

B irreversible alopecia

C opportunistic infection with a protozoon (eg pneumocystis)

D urate nephropathy, preventable by allopurinol

E a temporary mutagenic effect on gonadal cells

38.8 **Adverse effects of anticancer drugs include**

A occurrence of lymphoma five years after treatment

B risk to pregnant health staff from handling drugs

C production of a drug aerosol on opening an ampoule

D bone marrow depression

E male sterility

38.9 **In hormone-dependent cancer**

A adrenocortical hormones, though useful for complications, have no direct action on the cancer itself

B prostate cancer is androgen-dependent

C breast cancer is less likely to respond to oophorectomy in postmenopausal than in premenopausal women

D a better therapeutic result in breast cancer can be attained in tumours having both oestrogen and progesterone receptors

E tamoxifen confers no benefit on postmenopausal women with breast cancer

38.10 **The following statements about cytotoxic agents are correct:**

A Alkylating agents interfere with normal DNA synthesis
B Methotrexate competitively inhibits dihydrofolate reductase
C Folinic acid (calcium leucovorin) terminates the action of methotrexate
D Fluorouracil is a purine antagonist
E Azathioprine is a pyrimidine antagonist

38.11 **In the field of cytotoxic agents**

A radiophosphorus is the treatment of choice for polycythaemia vera
B side-effects may be so severe that patients refuse therapy
C vincristine causes cell cycle arrest
D antibiotics such as bleomycin interfere with DNA/RNA synthesis
E it is now generally agreed that laetrile can relieve pain and prolong survival

38.12 **Tumours in which significant benefit is common and life expectancy may become normal after chemotherapy include**

A multiple myeloma
B oropharyngeal carcinoma
C seminoma
D squamous bronchial carcinoma
E lymphoma

38.13 **One of the first choice drugs for**

A chronic granulocytic leukaemia is busulphan
B Hodgkin's lymphoma is cyclophosphamide
C brain cancer is procarbazine
D ovary cancer is doxorubicin
E choriocarcinoma is actinomycin D

38.14 **In immunosuppressive treatment**

A   established immunity is suppressed more readily than the development of an immune response after antigenic challenge

B   cyclosporin selectively inhibits multiplication of the immunocompetent T-lymphocyte

C   response to a non-living poliomyelitis vaccine is diminished

D   its hazards in rheumatoid arthritis are more acceptable in young people

E   antilymphocytic globulin does not induce allergy

39 Drugs and Skin

39.1 When a drug is applied to the skin

A absorption is greater if an occlusive dressing is used
B healing of untreated distant lesions may occur
C it is of little importance what vehicle is used
D the consequences vary with the state of the keratin layer
E it cannot enter the deeper layers of the skin through hair follicles

39.2 Lotions

A are contraindicated in acutely inflamed lesions
B are less useful if there is much exudation
C exert their soothing effect through the evaporation of water
D are less often used than are creams in the alleviation of pruritus
E can reduce body temperature dangerously in old people

39.3 The following statements about skin creams are correct:

A An emulsion such as Zinc Cream mixes with serous discharges
B Water-in-oil emulsions are more easy to spread than ointments
C Water repellent barrier creams are highly effective in preventing occupational dermatitis
D Silicone sprays are useful in the prevention and treatment of pressure sores
E Masking creams are used mostly to protect against sunburn

39.4 In the therapy of skin disease

A non-emulsifying preparations such as Paraffin Ointment are particularly useful to deliver active agents on hairy areas
B pastes are ointments containing insoluble powders
C Zinc Starch and Talc Dusting-powder is likely to increase friction between skin surfaces
D insect repellents such as dimethylphthalate remain effective even in the presence of profuse sweating
E keratolytics may damage normal skin as well as soften horny layers

39.5 An alcoholic solution of chlorhexidine

A disinfects the hands if rubbed on till dry
B is the most suitable preparation for the disinfection of stainless steel objects
C is the disinfectant of choice preoperatively if diathermy is to be used
D is essential as a preliminary to venepuncture
E provides the best treatment for impetigo

39.6 The following statements about antiseptics are correct:

A 100% alcohol penetrates and kills microbes more effectively than 70% alcohol
B Hexachlorophane is toxic to the central nervous system if absorbed through the skin
C Povidine-iodine has no antibacterial action in the presence of blood or exudate
D Hydrogen peroxide has a useful mechanical action as well as being a weak antimicrobial
E Cetrimide is a cationic surfactant

39.7 In the treatment of skin infections

A tetracycline combined with adrenal steroid is commonly used in children with infected eczema

B neomycin ointment may be absorbed in sufficient quantity to cause deafness if used on large areas

C if nystatin is used as an antifungal agent it must be given systemically

D an allergic reaction commonly occurs with the use of penicillin on the skin

E topical malathion is best given for pediculosis as a lotion

39.8 Itching, when its cause is unknown or unremovable, may be alleviated by

A Methyl Salicylate Ointment

B prostaglandins

C phenol

D aspirin

E crotamiton

39.9 When an adrenocorticosteroid preparation is used in skin disease

A systemic treatment should only be given in a serious condition such as pemphigus

B topical application does not allow sufficient absorption to cause systemic toxicity

C abrupt withdrawal does not exacerbate disease

D a potent fluorinated steroid is first choice for eczema

E skin atrophy and striae may follow local application

39.10 Photosensitivity

A may be produced by oral contraceptives

B sometimes follows the local use of deodorants

C can result in the inhibition of DNA and RNA synthesis and the release of prostaglandins

D can be prevented by the regular use of dihydroxyacetone

E in porphyria is best controlled by oral chloroquine

39.11 Drugs given systemically may cause

A erythema multiforme
B erythema nodosum
C exfoliative dermatitis
D chronic urticaria
E hair loss

39.12 Dermal adverse reactions

A to systemically administered drugs are commonly erythematous
B due to local contact are nearly always urticarial
C are usually of the same kind in all patients who take the offending drug
D recur at the same site in fixed eruptions
E usually only occur after a drug has been taken for months

39.13 Psoriasis

A can be rationally treated with oestrogen-containing creams
B is associated with increased numbers of horn cells containing abnormal keratin
C of the scalp is often treated by tar preparations
D can sometimes be helped by psoralens
E is unresponsive to adrenal steroids

39.14 In the treatment of acne

A frequent skin cleansing and degreasing is sufficient for milder cases
B isotretinoin should only be used in the most severe cases because it is a teratogen
C tetracycline suppresses the bacterial lipolysis of sebum
D there is no place for an antiandrogen such as cyproterone
E benzoyl peroxide unblocks pilosebaceous ducts

39.15 Adrenal steroids have a place in the treatment of

A alopecia areata
B seborrhoeic dermatitis
C herpes simplex
D rosacea
E dermatitis herpetiformis

39.16 The following statements are correct:

A Nappy rash is treated by a detergent such as cetrimide
B Oestrogen-containing creams are of great value in the treatment of acne
C There is no effective treatment for scleroderma
D Warts often disappear spontaneously
E Chemical depilatories make hair fibres jellify so that they can be wiped off

40 Vitamins, Calcium, Bone

40.1 Vitamin A deficiency

A is to be expected in strict vegetarians
B causes night blindness
C is relatively common in Asia
D should be thought of in a case of steatorrhoea
E causes epithelial metaplasia

40.2 The B group of vitamins

A are soluble in water
B are concerned in essential oxidation-reduction reactions
C are present in meat and yeast
D are not synthesised in any way in the body
E are needed by patients maintained on intravenous feeding for more than two days

40.3 Thiamine deficiency

A is not usually accompanied by other vitamin deficiency
B should be considered in any case of obscure peripheral neuropathy
C may result in high output cardiac failure
D is likely to occur in populations who eat a staple diet of brown rice
E is accompanied by the accumulation of pyruvic and other α-keto-acids

40.4 The following statements about B vitamins are correct:

A Riboflavine deficiency causes vascularisation of the cornea
B Dementia occurs as a result of nicotinamide deficiency
C Pellagra is less likely to occur in an underfed population if maize is the staple food
D Pyridoxine can block the therapeutic effect of levodopa in parkinsonism
E Despite its capacity to activate cystathionine synthetase, pyridoxine is of no value in the treatment of homocystinuria

40.5 Vitamin C deficiency

A can be prevented equally effectively by all citrus fruits
B causes bleeding gums in old people especially if they are edentulous
C manifested as scurvy does not occur in any animal other than man
D results in delayed wound healing
E is more likely to occur in babies fed on cows' milk than on breast milk

40.6 Methaemoglobinaemia

A impairs the oxygen carrying capacity of the blood
B may be due to treatment with sulphonamides
C is better treated in urgent cases with ascorbic acid than by methylene blue
D can occur in a congenital form
E responds less well to treatment than does sulphaemoglobinaemia

40.7　In tetany

A　hysterical overbreathing is a common cause
B　aluminium hydroxide by mouth binds phosphate in the gut
　　and indirectly enhances calcium absorption
C　a feeling of warmth spreading over the body after
　　intravenous calcium has been given is a sign of danger
D　cholecalciferol acts more quickly than dihydrotachysterol
E　the use of parathormone is limited by the development of
　　immunological resistance

40.8　Acute hypercalcaemia is benefited by

A　controlled dehydration
B　frusemide
C　prednisolone
D　mithramycin if the cause is bone cancer
E　oral phosphate

40.9　Calcitonin

A　is a steroid hormone
B　is produced in the thymus remnant
C　enhances the rate of bone turnover
D　increases renal tubular absorption of calcium and
　　phosphorus
E　is used to control hypercalcaemia

40.10　The following statements about vitamin D are correct:

A　Alfacalcidol is superior to cholecalciferol because it does
　　not require renal hydroxylation to become active
B　Dihydrotachysterol is similar in its effects to alfacalcidol
C　Calcium with Vitamin D Tabs contain approximately the
　　same amount of vitamin D as Calciferol Tabs High-strength
D　A large single dose of vitamin D has biological effects for
　　as long as six months
E　Epileptics on long term anticonvulsant therapy are prone
　　to vitamin D deficiency

40.11 The pain of Paget's disease of bone may be relieved by

   A improving the blood supply with tocopherols
   B inhibiting bone resorption with calcitonin
   C inhibiting crystal formation with diphosphonate
   D inhibiting osteoclasts with a cytotoxic agent
   E increasing osteocyte activity with parathormone

Answers

Chapter 1

Question	Answer
1	BDE
2	ABCDE
3	BCD
4	AD
5	B
6	AC
7	ABD
8	DE
9	ADE
10	ABCD
11	B
12	ABDE
13	ABCDE
14	BCDE
15	E
16	C
17	ACD
18	CDE
19	ABCDE
20	ABCDE
21	BC
22	AE

Chapter 2

1	ABD

Chapter 3

1	AE
2	CDE
3	CDE
4	DE

Chapter 4

1	ABCDE
2	ADE
3	C

Chapter 4 (contd)

Question	Answer
4	B
5	C
6	ABCDE
7	ABD
8	ABE
9	BCD
10	ABCE
11	BC
12	CE
13	BE
14	ABCDE

Chapter 5

1	ABD
2	ABCDE
3	ABCDE
4	AC
5	BE
6	ADE

Chapter 6

1	ABC
2	CDE
3	E

Chapter 7

1	BCDE
2	ABCE

Chapter 8

1	ABCDE
2	ACDE
3	CDE
4	AC
5	ABC
6	E

Chapter 8 (contd)

Question	Answer
7	ABD
8	BCD
9	ACD
10	BCE
11	ACE
12	ABCE
13	ABCDE
14	ABC
15	BCDE
16	ABDE
17	ABCE
18	ABE
19	ACD
20	ABCDE
21	ABCE
22	ADE
23	ACDE
24	ABCE
25	ABE
26	C
27	BCE
28	ABCDE
29	BCDE
30	ABCD
31	ABCD
32	CDE
33	ABCDE
34	ABC
35	A
36	AB
37	ABCE
38	BC
39	ABCDE
40	CDE
41	E
42	ABCDE
43	CE
44	BCD
45	DE

Question	Answer
1	BCD
2	ABCDE
3	BDE
4	CDE
5	BE
6	BCE
7	C
8	ABCDE
9	ABCE
10	CDE
11	BCE
12	ABCE
13	ABCE
14	CE
15	CE
16	CE
17	BDE
18	ABDE
19	ABCDE
20	C
21	ABCE
22	ABD
23	ACDE
24	BCD
25	BCDE
26	ABCDE

Chapter 10

Question	Answer
1	CE
2	ABE
3	AD
4	ACE
5	ABE
6	BDE
7	ABCDE
8	AC
9	ACD
10	AD
11	BDE
12	AD
13	ABCDE

Chapter 11

Question	Answer
1	CE
2	ABE
3	AE
4	ABC
5	ACDE
6	ABCDE
7	ABCDE

Chapter 12

Question	Answer
1	AD
2	AE
3	ABD
4	ABCD
5	BCDE
6	BDE
7	ACDE
8	ABCD
9	BCDE
10	ACD
11	ABC
12	ABCDE
13	ACD

Chapter 13

Question	Answer
1	CD
2	B
3	ABC
4	ABC
5	BCD
6	ABDE
7	BE
8	AC
9	CD
10	ABC
11	DE
12	ABC
13	BCE
14	ABCE
15	ABDE
16	ABCE
17	ABD
18	BE

Chapter 14

Question	Answer
1	ABCDE
2	AD
3	BC
4	BE
5	BCD
6	ACDE
7	BE

Chapter 15

Question	Answer
1	ABCDE
2	CD
3	BCDE
4	DE
5	ABCE
6	ACDE
7	CDE
8	ACD
9	BCDE
10	ABC
11	ABE

Chapter 16

Question	Answer
1	AE
2	ABCDE
3	DE
4	BCDE
5	B
6	ABE
7	ABD
8	CE
9	ABE
10	ABCE
11	BDE
12	ABCDE
13	AD
14	ABCDE
15	AE
16	ABCDE
17	BCDE
18	ABC
19	C
20	ACDE
21	CDE

Chapter 16 (contd)

Question	Answer
22	D
23	ABCDE
24	BCDE
25	ABE
26	BD

Chapter 17

Question	Answer
1	ABCDE
2	ABE
3	CDE
4	CDE
5	B
6	C
7	AE
8	BCE
9	C
10	ABCE
11	ACE

Chapter 18

Question	Answer
1	ACDE
2	ABC
3	CE
4	ABDE
5	D
6	ABCDE
7	CDE
8	ABDE
9	ABCDE
10	ABDE
11	BCD
12	BCD
13	ABCDE
14	BCE
15	BD
16	E
17	BCDE
18	BCDE
19	CE
20	ACDE

Chapter 19

Question	Answer
1	BDE
2	ACDE
3	AE
4	ABD
5	C
6	BCDE
7	AD
8	BDE
9	ABCE
10	BCD
11	D
12	ABCD
13	ABCE
14	BC
15	BC
16	CDE

Chapter 20

Question	Answer
1	ABCDE
2	ACDE
3	BD
4	CDE
5	ABCDE
6	BDE
7	ACE
8	D
9	ACD
10	ACDE
11	BC
12	ABCDE
13	ACE
14	ABCD
15	ABCE
16	ABCDE
17	ABCDE
18	A
19	CE
20	AB
21	BDE
22	CE
23	ABCDE
24	ACE
25	ABD
26	BE

Chapter 20 (contd)

Question	Answer
27	D
28	ACDE
29	ABE
30	BCD

Chapter 21

Question	Answer
1	AE
2	C
3	BCE
4	DE
5	ABC
6	BCE
7	ABDE
8	CE
9	ABD
10	ABCD
11	BD
12	AB
13	AD
14	BDE
15	CD
16	ACD
17	ABC
18	DE
19	BCE
20	ABCD
21	AD
22	ABDE
23	BDE
24	B
25	BCD
26	ABCDE
27	ABCD

Chapter 22

Question	Answer
1	AD
2	ABDE
3	BE
4	ABCD
5	ABE
6	ACE
7	ABCD
8	AC

Question	Answer
9	ADE
10	ABDE
11	ABCDE

Chapter 23

Question	Answer
1	ABE
2	ABCDE
3	ABD
4	C
5	BCDE
6	DE
7	ABCD
8	ADE
9	ABCDE
10	ABCD
11	ABCD

Chapter 24

Question	Answer
1	ABDE
2	BCDE
3	AE
4	CD
5	ABE
6	AB
7	ACE
8	B
9	ACD
10	BDE
11	BE
12	ABCE
13	CE
14	ABCDE
15	ACDE
16	BCD
17	BCD
18	ABDE
19	ABCDE
20	ABCE
21	BCE
22	BDE
23	ABDE
24	ABCE
25	D

Question	Answer
26	ABC
27	BCD
28	BCDE
29	BCE
30	CDE

Chapter 25

Question	Answer
1	ACE
2	A
3	ABCE
4	ABDE
5	ABE
6	ABE
7	ABD
8	BDE
9	BD
10	CDE
11	CDE
12	ABD
13	AB
14	E
15	BD
16	ABDE
17	ADE
18	BC
19	ACDE
20	ACE
21	ABDE
22	DE
23	ABCD
24	ACD

Chapter 26

Question	Answer
1	BDE
2	CDE

Chapter 27

Question	Answer
1	BC
2	ABC
3	C
4	E
5	AD

Question	Answer
6	BCDE
7	ABDE
8	ABDE
9	ABC
10	ACE
11	ABCE
12	ABDE
13	ABDE
14	CD
15	ABD
16	BDE
17	ABCD
18	ABCE
19	BCDE
20	ABC
21	ABCDE
22	ABCD
23	AB
24	ABCD
25	BCD
26	E
27	CE

Chapter 28

Question	Answer
1	ABDE
2	ABE
3	ACD
4	BC
5	DE
6	ABCE
7	BDE
8	ABE
9	ADE
10	BE
11	BDE
12	ABCE
13	D

Chapter 29

Question	Answer
1	DE
2	ABDE
3	AC
4	BCDE

Question	Answer
5	CE
6	ADE
7	BE
8	CDE
9	CE

Chapter 30

1	ABC
2	CDE
3	BCE
4	ABE
5	BE
6	ABCDE
7	ABCD
8	ABCD
9	ABCDE
10	BDE
11	ACE
12	D
13	ACDE
14	ABD
15	ABCD

Chapter 31

1	A
2	ABDE
3	BCD
4	ABC
5	BDE

Chapter 32

1	BC
2	ABCE
3	ABCDE
4	BCE
5	AD
6	BCE
7	BCD
8	ABCDE
9	ABDE
10	BCDE
11	ABD

Question	Answer
12	ABE
13	BCD
14	ACDE

Chapter 33

1	D
2	CE
3	BCD

Chapter 34

1	BDE
2	ABC
3	B
4	A
5	ADE
6	BCD
7	BC
8	ACDE
9	AD
10	BDE
11	ABCE
12	ACDE
13	BDE
14	AE
15	ABDE
16	BC
17	ACE
18	ACE
19	ABCDE
20	CE
21	B
22	ABCDE
23	ABCE
24	ACDE
25	CDE
26	ABCDE
27	ABDE
28	BD
29	ACDE

Chapter 35

1	ABE

Question	Answer
2	ACDE
3	BCD
4	BCE
5	ABCE
6	AB
7	BD
8	BCE
9	D
10	ABCDE
11	CDE
12	BCE

Chapter 36

1	ABCDE
2	ABCE
3	A
4	ABCD
5	ABCE
6	AB
7	ADE
8	AC

Chapter 37

1	AD
2	BCD
3	ABCE
4	AE
5	CD
6	ABD
7	ABCD
8	ABD
9	BCD
10	BC
11	AC
12	ABCD
13	ACDE
14	A
15	CD
16	BC
17	BD
18	BCDE
19	CE

Chapter 38		Chapter 39		Chapter 40	
Question	Answer	Question	Answer	Question	Answer
1	ABD	1	ABD	1	BCDE
2	BCDE	2	CE	2	ABCE
3	AE	3	BD	3	BCE
4	BE	4	BE	4	ABD
5	CD	5	A	5	DE
6	ABD	6	BDE	6	ABD
7	ACDE	7	ABDE	7	ABCE
8	ABCDE	8	CDE	8	BCDE
9	BCD	9	AE	9	E
10	ABC	10	ABC	10	ABDE
11	ABC	11	ABCDE	11	BCD
12	CE	12	AD		
13	ABD	13	BCD		
14	BC	14	ABCE		
		15	BE		
		16	CDE		